Yoga
for
Arthritis

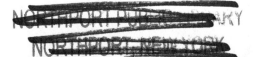

Yoga for Arthritis

THE COMPLETE GUIDE

Loren M. Fishman, MD, BPhil, (oxon.)

Ellen Saltonstall, MA

W. W. Norton & Company

New York • London

For information about permission to reproduce selections from this book,
write to Permissions, W. W. Norton & Company, Inc.,
500 Fifth Avenue, New York, NY 10110

For information about special discounts for bulk purchases, please contact
W. W. Norton Special Sales at specialsales@wwnorton.com or 800-233-4830

Manufacturing by Courier Westford
Book design by Molly Heron
Production manager: Devon Zahn

Library of Congress Cataloging-in-Publication Data

Fishman, Loren.
Yoga for arthritis : the complete guide / Loren M. Fishman,
Ellen Saltonstall. — 1st ed.
p. cm.
Includes bibliographical references and index.
ISBN 978-0-393-33058-8 (pbk.)
1. Arthritis—Exercise therapy. 2. Yoga—Therapeutic use.
I. Saltonstall, Ellen. II. Title.
RC933.F543 2008
616.7'220642—dc22

2007044693

W. W. Norton & Company, Inc.
500 Fifth Avenue, New York, N.Y. 10110
www.wwnorton.com

W. W. Norton & Company Ltd.
Castle House, 75/76 Wells Street, London W1T 3QT

1 2 3 4 5 6 7 8 9 0

DEDICATION

To all the yoga teachers, physicians, and true healers who have taught their craft, who have handed down their knowledge and kept it alive from preliterate times, and who are doing so now.

CONTENTS

LIST OF ILLUSTRATIONS

LIST OF TABLES

For the aid of therapists, the actions of poses are tabulated
at the end of each chapter.

ACKNOWLEDGMENTS

We are grateful to our revered teachers, B. K. S. Iyengar and John Friend, and many others for their patient teaching and spontaneous inspiration; to Diva Robinson and Denna Reilly, our co-models; Donal Holway and Julio Torres for their fine-sensed and reliably good judgment in doing the photography; Susan Genis, Bindu Wiles, Sally Hess, and Tova Ovadia for their discerning eyes and practical suggestions; Carol Stratten, Dr. David Palmieri, Dr. Allan Cummings, and Norman Brettler for their work and help with dynamic MRI studies; Mary Ann Dunkin of the Arthritis Foundation for all her help; Jill Bialosky and Evan Carver for unfailing trust and continued editorial support; our students and patients for all they have taught us; and our families for their articulate silence and kind forebearance while we were not there.

AUTHORS' NOTE

One of the chief differences between sciences and religions is that sciences cooperate with one another. Since all truth is necessarily consistent, no true statement can be a contradiction of any other. Therefore, Darwin used the work of geologists and biologists equally. Watson and Crick depended on X-ray crystallography, and Newton had recourse to optics in his work on gravity.

Religions, alas, do not have this unanimous acceptance of one another's truth. A striking example may be the three Western monotheistic religions, which define one god as the creator of the universe and thus are in total agreement. There could not be more than one such creator, so it follows that they all worship the very same being. Nevertheless, no one could mistake the historical or current situation for the unanimity that this implies. Europe was in flames for hundreds of years in the name of the Prince of Peace. This day, explosions will likely murder or maim innocent people who believe the vast majority of what their attackers do. We may ask after the basis of loyalty to a leader who revives hate based on small differences rather than use his or her life-force to lay bare our commonality.

Without resorting to physical violence, yoga is in danger of slipping into the same sort of factionalism.

It is our intent in this book to merge together somewhat different traditions, yogic and scientific. Our goal is to find (and to encourage other people to search for) what is most helpful for our fellow beings, based on all peoples' similarities as described by science. While there is certainly room for individual preference, there is nothing discretionary about the truth. We hope that this book, based on our inherently limited experience and ideas, will be of some value, and that its many flaws will serve to stimulate others to do better.

Most skills represent an internalization of what was once a consciously learned practice. Painters' "second nature" is to follow their rules of composition, drummers deftly hold the sticks just so, experienced debaters almost unconsciously shape a phrase. Yoga is somewhat the opposite. Yogis may slow their hearts, work to regulate their breathing, and bring up to consciousness and refine what was mastered and became "automatic" as an infant. People can perform yoga poses like trained seals perform their tricks, having learned "what to do," but it is not exactly what Patanjali, author of the *Yoga Sutra*, or alert contemporary practitioners have in mind. Yoga promotes familiarity with the unconscious factors within the mind in order to master them.

In Classical Yoga, in order to gain control over the mind, one moves and manipulates the body. By using what is outside—heart rate, breaths, posture—to gain control of what is inside—thoughts and emotions—yoga has launched a Copernican revolution of great promise. Later developments in yoga recognize the beauty and capacity of the human spirit as it manifests in everyday life, and teach us to experience that through the disciplined practice of yoga. We have been inspired by B. K. S. Iyengar, who has discovered, perfected, or totally created hundreds of poses. John Friend, the founder of Anusara Yoga, has analyzed these and added his own principles, to form an almost axiomatic approach. But despite the science we explain in this book, yoga itself is not a science. An individual may pick a type of yoga or a teacher for aesthetic, cultural, or personal reasons, or for convenience, because of one's friends or parents, or the persuasive power of a book, and any of these reasons is acceptable. In this respect, the schools of yoga are like contemporaneous movements in art: Dadaism living alongside Impressionism, Neoclassicism, and the Bauhaus. The simile is limited, though, since movements in art are often directly and explicitly opposed to one another, and aimed at replacing the ones that precede them. But any free society encourages this diversity.

In a sense, the happy diversity of schools of yoga is like freedom of religion: every religion is equally welcome, provided it, like the others, has a common belief in the perfectibility of man, the desire for peace, and the right of other religions to thrive. Jacob Burckhardt wrote of religion: "Now, no religion has ever been quite independent of the culture of its people and its time. It is just when . . . it is interwoven with life as a whole that life will most infallibly react upon it."[1] Though yoga is emphatically not a religion, but simply a practice, it too intends to be "interwoven with life as a whole." One example of yoga's integration is mixed-gender classes, which were unthinkable a hundred years ago and are still shunned in some parts of the world. Another is the possibly more serious contact between yoga and contemporary science.

Since we have yet to see the first scientific comparison of one style of yoga with another, it seems reasonable to assume that we choose a style more or less the way we choose a religion: aesthetics, family, friends, personal preferences, the charisma of a given proponent. Therefore, it makes little sense to trumpet one's own preference as "better for you" or "the right one for arthritis" (or cancer, or depression, etc.) until that has been shown to be true. Whatever else yoga may be, it is allied with the wisdom of men and women of old in every land—Indian, Greek, Chinese, and Native American: to choose the rational course, however iconoclastic to the dominant mores of their own people. It would be antithetical to the whole idea of yoga to close-mindedly contend that simply because we believe something, it is the closest we can come to the truth.

We now have the means, with science, to determine what is good for what, and why. We can suffer the unfortunate fate of so many religions and maintain the supremacy of what we happen to believe, in spite of its being absolutely unsupported by a single empirical observation,[2] or we can open our eyes and confirm or refute our current beliefs.

It is amazing that the great monotheistic religions of the world, though they all believe in a single creator of the universe, fail to coexist and cooperate. If yoga is going to grow in usefulness, physicians, yogis, and scientists must communicate in an atmosphere of mutual respect.

We happen to stand at the perimeter of a vast and well-kept clearing. It is the intersection of two great thoroughfares of thought, medicine and yoga, each many centuries in the making. One edge of the clearing may be empirical, another may be spiritual. The clearing is so great, compared to our capacity for sensing and understanding, that from one side we cannot easily see to the other. We can stubbornly claim one small part of it as our own, and diligently defend its boundaries. Or we can explore.

Yoga
for
Arthritis

INTRODUCTION

Serendipitously or not, arthritis and yoga fit: the lock and the key, the illness and the antidote. Arthritis restricts movement, yoga increases range of motion—these two were made for each other. The inevitable pounding, flexing, and grinding the human body experiences during life have pressured it to evolve many anatomical cushions, but alas, they too inevitably suffer from life's buffeting. The incessant minor traumas add up, damaging the cushioning apparatus and eventually the structures they protect, increasing pain and instability, and reducing flexibility at the only places we can bend: the joints. Yoga has been shown to improve the microenvironment of the cartilage and elastic parts of the joint and add no trauma. And for thousands of years it has been known to increase flexibility.

In this book we provide a scientific justification for using yoga to treat arthritis. It is intended for beginners, those already doing yoga, and teachers, yoga therapists, and other healers such as physical and occupational therapists and physicians. Therefore, it might approximate a one-room-schoolhouse atmosphere at times, addressing rank beginners and the accomplished yogi in the sincere voice of two authors who know some things fairly well, but know very well how very much is not known.

In the first two chapters, we familiarize you with arthritis the condition, and then yoga, the best we have found for prevention and relief. Next we present a science-oriented chapter on the physiology behind yoga's efficacy for arthritis. Then, after a short prelude, come the poses. At the end of each chapter we provide a table to aid therapists, healers, and individuals in designing a program for the particular difficulties a given person may present. Although we have successfully treated many patients with yoga alone, we believe it is only with rigorous objective testing that this modality can be proved and improved, and that combining yoga with other means of healing, conventional and not, will stand before the same objective scrutiny.

CHAPTER 1

Arthritis

What Is Arthritis?

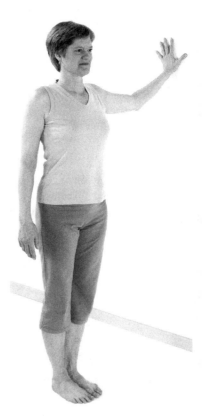

Age is not a disease. It is a state to which most of us aspire. But advancing years do not come without a price. For many of us, one price of a long life is osteoarthritis, a painful and often debilitating condition caused by decades of wear and tear on the joints. In fact, by the time we reach age sixty-five, knee X-rays for at least a third of us will show some signs of osteoarthritis,[1] the most common of a group of diseases collectively referred to simply as *arthritis*.

Literally translated "joint inflammation," arthritis in its many forms affects more than seventy million (or one in three) American adults, according to estimates by the Centers for Disease Control and Prevention in Atlanta. Arthritis is the leading cause of disability in this country, limiting everyday activities for more than seven million adults.[2]

Although the specifics of the different types of arthritis vary, they have a common thread: all affect the joints, those nearly 150 ingenious—and essential—structures located where two or more bones come together. With a few exceptions, these joints (when working properly) are easily movable, allowing us to bend, flex, sit, grasp, open and close our mouths, lift, turn, get out of bed, and walk—or run—where we need to go.

How Healthy Joints Work

In healthy joints, articular cartilage—a tough, shock-absorbing padding with a slick surface—enables the ends of the bones to glide effortlessly past each other. This gliding is facilitated by a viscous lubricating fluid (a natural WD-40, of sorts) called synovial fluid, which is secreted by a thin membrane, the synovium, that lines the joint. Bones are held together at the joints by strong, inelastic bands of tissue, called ligaments, that help keep the joint aligned. Tough cords of tissue, the tendons, connect muscle to bone. Muscles work in opposing pairs to bend and straighten joints. While muscles are not technically part of a joint, they are important because strong muscles help support and protect joints and cause bones to move. Outside the joints, fluid-filled sacs called bursae cushion and safely separate the bones and tendons around the joints, enabling them to move smoothly and freely.

What Goes Wrong in Osteoarthritis?

Osteoarthritis can be the result of so many different factors that it might often appear to have no identifiable cause. In a way, that is what people mean when they say it is due to "wear and tear." They mean that just living will lead to osteoarthritis.

We have already mentioned trauma and overuse as special cases where a cause *can* be identified. Deficiencies in the chemical structures that make up the cushions, the glycosaminoglycans, are another special cause. Many other genetic, hormonal, and environmental factors are also relevant: somatotropin C, growth hormone, thyroxine, testosterone, corticosteroids, and estrogen, to name a few.

Whereas osteoarthritis usually develops over time from the processes of wear and tear, factors such as a severe injury to the joint that damages the cartilage or throws off the alignment of the bones can cause cartilage to wear unevenly and start the osteoarthritis process earlier. Also, research has shown that some people have inherited defects in joint cartilage, such as Ehlers-Danlos syndrome and Marfan syndrome,

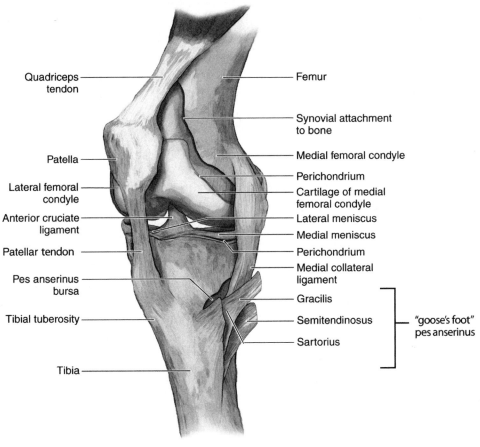

Quadriceps tendon

Femur

Synovial attachment to bone

Patella

Medial femoral condyle

Perichondrium

Lateral femoral condyle

Cartilage of medial femoral condyle

Anterior cruciate ligament

Lateral meniscus

Medial meniscus

Patellar tendon

Perichondrium

Pes anserinus bursa

Medial collateral ligament

Gracilis

Tibial tuberosity

Semitendinosus

Sartorius

"goose's foot" pes anserinus

Tibia

Anteromedial View

Figure 1. *A representative joint—the knee. The pes anserinus bursa is so named because the three tendons that join there resemble a goose's foot. Bursae separate bones from the muscles that cross them, protecting each from the other. Arthritic movement patterns, however, may inflame the bursae, causing pain exactly where they normally prevent it.*

that predispose them to the early development of osteoarthritis.[3,4] For our purposes—relieving the pain and limitation that come with arthritis—we focus on the actual sites of damage: the joints.

Over the course of a lifetime, the cartilage that covers the ends of the bones can begin to wear away. But cartilage is mainly inanimate—it is a lifeless product of live cells, like nails and hair. Just like hair, it is in continuous production. And just like nails, the distribution and condition of the underlying cells determine the quality and elasticity of the cartilage.

A good quantity of viscous lubricating fluid bathes the joint, making its movements smooth and easy. A capsule of connective tissue encloses the joint like a gasket, containing the joint fluid. Synovial cells at the inner surface of the capsule secrete the joint fluid. Another special layer of cells, the perichondrium, lies beneath the cartilage, between it and the bone. Replete with blood vessels, it serves to nourish the chondrocytes, the cartilage-producing cells that dwell within the cartilage. The cartilage itself has no blood vessels.[5]

Cartilage located elsewhere in the body—not at joints—has perichondrium on both sides. For example, in the windpipe, perichondrium lines the inside as well as the outside of the cartilage rings. In contrast, joint cartilage is supported only from beneath, from the bone it grows out of, not from above, not at the actual point of bone-to-bone contact. Joint cartilage has no inner layer of supportive cells. Yet the inner surface of the cartilage is what actually comes in contact with its counterpart on the other bone, the part that sustains the pressures of movement. This cartilage may be where the need for nourishment and the building blocks for repair is greatest!

The joint fluid brings the essential supplies for nourishment and repair to the chondrocytes. The inner lining of the joints (the synovial membrane) not only makes the fluid, but also delivers oxygen, glucose, proteins, and other necessities to that fluid and absorbs the products of their metabolism. The beauty is that the very movement that serves the joint's function also circulates the fluid that makes continued movement possible. Circulation is good for the joint.[6] As Arthur Abrahamson, former chairman of the Department of Physical Medicine and Rehabilitation at Albert Einstein College of Medicine, was fond of saying, "Function breeds function."

One thing that yoga does for sure is move the joints into extreme but safe positions, allowing the obscure corners and crevices of each joint to be awash with its lubricating, life-sustaining fluid.

Without good circulation of the synovial fluid, the smooth surfaces of cartilage can fall into states of disrepair. The chondrocytes will not keep up with the pace of normal wear and tear. Fibers of collagen, which are what give cartilage its elastic properties, are not replaced quickly enough, and soon the cartilage loses its supple resilience. The surfaces become rough and cracked, which leads to more wearing away. (Chapter 3 has more on this important subject.)

Naturally, other factors, including hormonal and hereditary factors, and the frequency, intensity, and pattern of use, overuse, and trauma, are at work here too. All of these elements can add up to enough of a departure from a joint's normal, or homeostatic, condition to produce

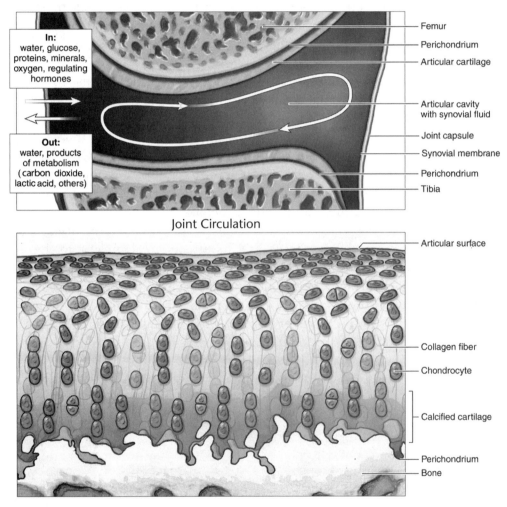

Joint Circulation

Close-up of Joint Cartilage

Figure 2. *Circulation of synovial fluid is critical to the well-being of cartilage. Joint movement through exercise is the only way to produce it.*

inflammation. It usually occurs without any infection, without anything actually breaking. This further compromises the cartilage, and actually stimulates the bone underlying it. In response to inflammation, and possibly in an effort to repair the damage, the ends of the bones might thicken and the bone might form outgrowths, called spurs or osteophytes, which can interfere with function and give the joint an enlarged, knobby appearance.

In joints between vertebrae at the cervical and lumbar levels, these osteophytes can obstruct the openings through which the nerves exit the spine, causing neurological signs and symptoms. The appropriate yoga for this lies in Chapters 8 and 9.

As cartilage is worn away, bone rubs more and more against bone. Pieces of cartilage and bone can break loose inside the joint, causing the joints to catch and to become stiff and noisy. If they are very active joints, such as the shoulders, or weight bearing, like the knees, this condition, known as chondrocalcinosis dessicans, can be extremely painful.

Osteoarthritis can affect a single joint or many. The most commonly affected joints are those of the knees, hips, neck, lower back, fingers, and the base of the thumb and big toe.

If anything good can be said for osteoarthritis, it is that the disease typically spares younger people and its effects are confined to the joints. With some other forms of arthritis, the debilitating effects can come during what should be the most productive years of life—the peak earning and child-rearing years—or even earlier. In addition to their effects on joints, some forms of arthritis can also cause damage to the skin, eyes, blood vessels, and internal organs.

The Other Forms of Arthritis

Let us take a look at some of the other more common forms of arthritis.

Rheumatoid Arthritis

Next to osteoarthritis, the most common form of arthritis is rheumatoid arthritis, affecting an estimated 2.1 million Americans.[7] Unlike osteoarthritis, which is largely a disease of mechanical wear and tear, rheumatoid arthritis is believed to be an autoimmune disease—that is, a disease in which the body's immune system turns against and destroys healthy tissue. In rheumatoid arthritis, the primary targets of the attack are the synovial linings of the joints and sometimes the similarly designed membranes lining the blood vessels, heart, and lungs.

In a joint affected by rheumatoid arthritis, both the synovial lining and the fluid it secretes become infiltrated with white blood cells from the lymph nodes, spleen, thymus, and circulating blood. These cells normally help protect the body from harmful invaders such as viruses, bacteria, and other microorganisms collectively known as antigens. But in rheumatoid arthritis a number of types of white blood cells can cause harm.

B cells (so named because they mature in the bone marrow) are responsible for the production of antibodies, proteins designed specifically to destroy a particular foreign substance. While antibodies help rid our bodies of infection, misdirected antibodies cause damage. Many people with rheumatoid arthritis have an abnormal antibody called rheumatoid factor (RF) in their blood. High levels of RF are generally associated with a more severe course of the disease. Other antibodies also target healthy tissue.

Mast cells, secreters of destructive enzymes, contribute to damage and dysfunction in both osteoarthritis and rheumatoid arthritis. Recently, they were found to occur in greater numbers in joints affected by osteoarthritis than in traumatically injured joints or even in joints with rheumatoid arthritis,[8] suggesting a special inflammatory role for them in osteoarthritis, and possibly another avenue for prevention and treatment in the future.

T cells (so named because they mature in the thymus) come in many forms. Some are responsible for helping B cells produce antibodies. Some are responsible for stopping the immune system's attack once the invader has been eliminated. Still others engulf and destroy antigen particles in the blood, destroy cell debris, or produce powerful chemical secretions that trigger or help regulate the body's immune response. They also present foreign material to the B cells for destruction, expediting the production of antibodies. In rheumatoid arthritis, some of this "foreign" material belongs to the person whose cells they are—not only is it not foreign, it is essential to the normal operation of the cell!

Macrophages are called scavenger cells because they clean up the mess left by B cells and T cells by eating up antigen particles left in the blood. They also secrete chemicals called cytokines that signal the immune system to either rev up or slow down its attack. In rheumatoid arthritis and many other forms of arthritis, a dysregulation of these chemicals and their signals contributes to symptoms and damage.

Neutrophils are white blood cells that fight infection and produce powerful enzymes that break down cell debris in the blood. These enzymes can be so virulent, in fact, that they can damage the synovial membranes that line the joints, and the cartilage that cushions them. Neutrophils also produce substances that increase blood flow to the affected area. Increased blood flow and internal fluids cause the affected joints to swell, and deliver other white blood cells that take part in the damaging attack, generally known as inflammation.

Unless the immune system's attack is stopped, rheumatoid arthritis can progress to damage not only the synovium but also the joint cartilage, underlying bone, and ligaments and tendons, causing deformity and disability.

The Spondyloarthropathies

Rather than a single form of arthritis, the spondylarthropathies comprise a group of diseases that affect the spine, the sacroiliac joints (where the lower end of the spine attaches to the pelvis), and the structures that join ligaments and tendons to bone. These diseases can also affect other joints, such as those of the arms, legs, feet, and hands, and body tissues, including the skin, eyes, bowel, and genitourinary tract.

It is estimated that between 354,000 and 412,000 Americans over age fifteen have a spondylarthropathy.[9] Following are the most common of these diseases.

Ankylosing spondylitis Largely a disease of young men, ankylosing spondylitis usually begins gradually with back pain, which can range

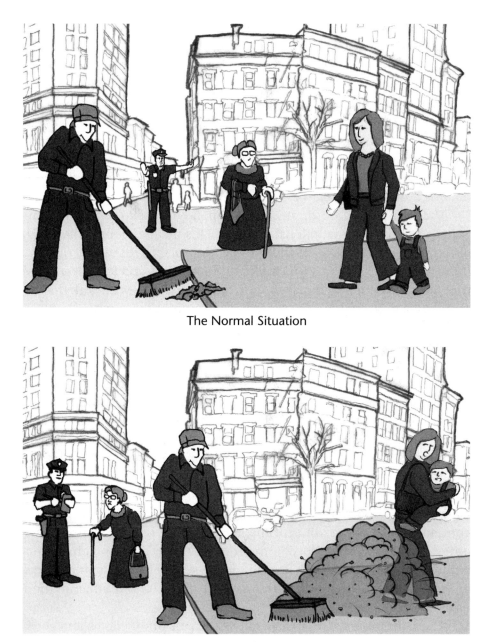

The Normal Situation

Rheumatoid Arthritis

Figure 3. *In rheumatoid arthritis the immune system retains its potency, but it performs its lethal tasks on the very cells it normally defends.*

from mild to severe and is generally worse at night or first thing in the morning. Some people also have pain that radiates down the legs.

Ankylosing spondylitis typically begins with inflammation around the sacroiliac joints, which might then progress up the spine. The ligaments and tendons that keep the bones of the spine in place and attach the muscles to the limbs and ribs can turn to bone, or ossify, causing the spine to become stiff or even rigid. In advanced cases, the spine may become fused into a stooped position, making bending or even turning the head impossible. The chest wall may also become rigid, making it difficult to breathe.

The treatment goal for ankylosing spondylitis is to reduce inflammation and to retain functional abilities. This means keeping the joints of the spine as flexible as possible and, if the spine is fused into rigidity, maximizing the flexibility and strength of the arms and legs. Good posture is important. It is also important for people with ankylosing spondylitis to strengthen the muscles that support the spine.

Reactive arthritis Also called Reiter's syndrome, reactive arthritis is so named because it occurs in reaction to an infection in another part of the body, typically the intestines, or kidneys, bladder, and genitals. For many people, reactive arthritis is preceded by a bout of diarrhea. It can also occur following urethritis (inflammation of the tube leading from the bladder through the penis that transports and discharges urine and semen) in men or cystitis (inflammation of the bladder) in women.

Reactive arthritis is characterized by inflammation of the joints as well as the surrounding ligaments, tendons, and muscles. It most commonly affects the joints of the legs and feet, but it can also affect other joints, including those of the fingers. Other common characteristics of the disease include a rash on the soles of the feet and palms of the hands, sores in the mouth or on the genitals, and inflammation of the eyes.

The joint inflammation of reactive arthritis often comes and goes. For some people the disease is chronic. In others it resolves and disappears completely over time. It represents another example of the immune system gone awry, this time initiated by an infection, a perfectly legitimate arousal of the body's immune defenses.

Psoriatic arthritis Psoriatic arthritis is a form of arthritis that affects 23 percent of people who have the skin disease psoriasis, according to the Psoriasis Foundation's 2001 Benchmark Survey.[10]

As with other forms of arthritis, psoriasis might be mediated by the immune system. However, recent evidence in experimental mice suggests that a certain part of chromosome 19, JunB, might be mutant or deleted in people with this disease.[11] These genes are known to regulate the speed of reproduction and stress response of the deeper layers of skin, and deleting the gene sequence in mice actually produced the signs and symptoms of psoriasis.

A normal skin cell matures and falls off the body's surface in twenty-eight to thirty days. But a psoriatic skin cell takes only three to four days to mature and move to the surface. Instead of falling off, the psoriatic cells pile up and form lesions. Depending on the specific form of psoriasis, the lesions can be raised and scaly, dotlike, intensely red and inflamed, or weeping.

In joints the disease process is a little more complicated, since both T cells and B cells play a role. It is likely that the immune system is somehow out of control here too.[12] Contemporary research suggests that in normal development, macrophages actually mark "extra" cells for death, and it is possible that this mechanism is working too hard in hereditary autoimmune illnesses as well.[13]

In addition to the joints of the spine, the arthritis that accompanies psoriasis can affect the fingers, toes, knees, and ankles. Psoriatic arthritis is similar to rheumatoid arthritis in that it is the body's own protective elements, the skin and the immune system, that do it ill. But psoriatic arthritis is generally milder. In psoriatic arthritis, the joints and the soft tissue around them become inflamed and stiff. However, severe psoriatic arthritis can be disabling and cause irreversible damage to joints.

Gout

Once associated with royalty, gout occurs when a bodily waste product called uric acid rises to such high levels in the bloodstream that it seeps out and deposits as sharp crystals in the joint tissue, much the way sugar settles to the bottom of a glass of iced tea. Uric acid is a result of the breakdown of purines, chemicals derived from nucleic acid in the cells. Many meats, especially organ meats, are high in purines. Your body also produces purines, which it then breaks down into uric acid.

Normally, the kidneys filter uric acid from the blood. Problems result when the body produces too much uric acid, or the kidneys cannot effectively eliminate excess uric acid.

Although gout can affect many joints—the feet, knees, elbows, and sometimes the finger and wrist joints—it typically begins with a single attack or periodic attacks in the big toe, a condition called podagra. During an attack, white blood cells rush to the joint, causing inflammation. The joint tissue swells and the skin over the joint becomes tight, shiny, and crimson. The pain can be excruciating. In his book *The Duke University Medical Center Book of Arthritis*, David Pisetsky writes, "One patient told me during an attack he noticed a housefly in the bedroom and couldn't take his eyes off that fly, terrified it would settle on his toe. Another worried that a piece of peeling paint from the ceiling was going to drop off on his toe."[14]

Gout affects an estimated 2.1 million Americans.[15] At middle age and younger, men are more likely than women to have gout. After menopause, the risk of developing gout for women is roughly that of men.

Unless gout is treated, attacks can become more frequent and severe and progress to affect more joints. For some people, fortunately, the proper diet (low in purine-rich foods and alcohol), exercise, and weight loss are effective at treating or even preventing the disease. In a twelve-year study of 47,150 men, doctors found that higher levels of meat and seafood consumption are associated with an increased risk of gout, whereas a higher level of consumption of dairy products is associated with a decreased risk.[16] A separate study of the same population showed that the risk of gout increased as body mass index increased. Men who lost ten pounds over the course of the twelve-year study cut their risk of gout almost in half, while those who gained thirty pounds since age twenty-one almost doubled their risk.[17]

Treating Arthritis

Advances in recent years have made it possible for people with many forms of arthritis to live longer, more productive, and less painful lives.

A variety of analgesics and nonsteroidal anti-inflammatory drugs (NSAIDs), available both over the counter and by prescription, help ease the pain of virtually any form of arthritis.

Strong immunosuppressive drugs or newer biological agents such as etanercept (Enbrel) and infliximab (Remicade) can help stop the disease processes of rheumatoid arthritis and the spondyloarthropathies. Corticosteroid medications such as prednisone and methylprednisolone (Medrol) can help halt inflammation that threatens the joints and internal organs in people with rheumatoid arthritis or other inflammatory forms of disease.

And for people with gout, anti-inflammatories (including NSAIDs), cochicine, corticosteroids, or adrenocorticotropic hormone (ACTH) can help ease the pain and inflammation of acute attacks, while other drugs that slow the production of uric acid or help the kidneys excrete it more efficiently can prevent—or at least lessen the frequency, duration, and severity of—future attacks.

When, despite the best medical treatment, joints are irreparably damaged and pain and stiffness limit daily activities, surgically replacing the joint with a prosthesis made of metal, plastic, or ceramic material can relieve pain and restore form and function.

Despite these treatment advances, which relieve pain, prevent damage, and preserve function, none is without a downside. Analgesics can become addictive. NSAIDs can cause stomach upset and ulcers, and recent reports show that some are not safe for our hearts.[18] Corticosteroids, though they are powerful against inflammation, can cause a wide range of problems, including weight gain, thin skin, cataracts, and brittle bones. Immunosuppressives and biological agents, too, have their downsides, ranging from injection-site reactions to increased risk of serious infections. Great advances? No doubt. Life saving? In some cases, yes. Perfect? Far from it.

Certainly there are cases where medications are necessary to control a disease that is threatening one's joints or even life. But relying on medication to the exclusion of other therapies and healthy lifestyle habits is a mistake. Study after study shows the benefits of exercise for many forms of arthritis. Exercise will improve strength and increase range of motion in affected joints. It will reduce the excess weight that contributes to the development of some forms of arthritis[19] and adds stress to painful joints. Exercise improves general well-being and mood and even etiolates signs of disease activity. This goes for many forms of arthritis, including osteoarthritis and gout.[20]

Then there is the combination of the two: medication and exercise. Although nonsteroidal and other medications do have side effects, and surely can be abused, there is little question of their beneficial influence on people suffering from arthritic disease. And they can be combined with yoga,[21] substantially amplifying the benefits of each. In some people, continued use of both is best; in others, medication can ease the pain and difficulty of beginning exercise, which, after a while, is sufficiently successful that it eliminates the need for medicines. In still others, medication and exercise can be used intermittently, as conditions permit and require.

In a progressively disabling condition such as arthritis, a multidisciplinary, integrative approach is quite effective; using everything available that is helpful, and avoiding overreliance on any one form of relief. Even with exercise there is that one caveat: don't overdo it. Exercise that is jarring or too strenuous can put stress on the joints and can make the problem worse, not better. That's why we recommend yoga.

Ready to give exercise a shot? Then let's get moving . . . gently.

CHAPTER 2

Yoga

Yoga has been practiced for thousands of years, its modern forms drawing on a very rich history of traditions and teachings. Its primary purpose has remained the same: to calm the mind and render it deeper and more subtle than our everyday awareness. As greater numbers of people worldwide turn to yoga for healing and personal growth, the vast dimension of what yoga has to offer can be eclipsed by its trendiness or by its flashier side—the calisthenics, the pretzel poses, the dramatic breathing techniques. People with arthritis might think, "I'm too stiff to do yoga" or "Yoga is too foreign and strange." In this book we make it clear that anyone can do yoga and gain a wide range of benefits.

The word *yoga* is derived from a Sanskrit root which means "to yoke or harness." On one level this can be taken to mean the harnessing of awareness, learning to focus the mind. Another level of meaning presupposes the notion of a supreme consciousness, an

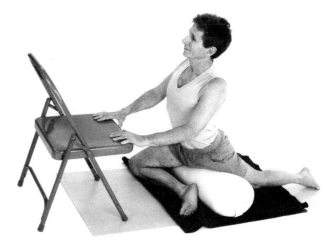

absolute reality, to which the individual spirit can be joined. Though its origins were clearly in the realms of spiritual discipline (possibly read "religion"), many people doing yoga today immerse themselves fully in the practice while still adhering to their own religious affiliations, agnosticism, or atheism.

As one writer put it, "Yoga itself is not a religion. It is undenominational, relying not on faith but on a number of techniques that gradually lead the individual to the direct experience of those truths on which religion rests. We can call it the inner spirit of religion."[1]

Although more than sixteen million Americans practice and believe in yoga,[2] it is nonsectarian. There is no organized "Church of Yoga," and likewise no faith we know of that opposes it. Classical yoga texts recognize a supreme being, but personal evolution is always the process and the goal. To be a student of yoga you must do yoga, that is all there is to it. Once you start it, the process is self-directing.

Yoga is often compared to a tree, with roots reliably traced at least as far back as to 2600 years BCE,[3] a strong trunk, and many branches that are still growing. If you go to a yoga class today, and when you do what is described in this book, you will be practicing a branch of the tree known as Hatha Yoga, the system of physical exercises that strengthen and stretch the body. The word *Hatha* refers to balancing opposite forces in the body. Within Hatha Yoga are many styles that have been developed by leading teachers; what we offer in this book is inspired directly by both Iyengar Yoga and Anusara Yoga, but it originated in antiquity. These styles are within the mainstream of yoga's long tradition but contain contemporary innovations informed by them.

Do we have to forego Western medical treatment in order to practice yoga? Absolutely not. The impressive accomplishments of Western medicine are built on the rational and empirical bases of Islamic, Indian, Greek, and Chinese medicine. Yet the West has turned more and more intently to the Eastern ways of life, and Western medicine has an ever-growing interest in Eastern methods of treatment and cure. We believe there are three major explanations for this trend. First, our expanding familiarity with the great world around us has quite naturally led those of us for whom conventional medical treatment is not successful to seek respected types of care from farther afield. Second, the impersonal corporatization of medicine has led many of us to seek more intimate one-to-one contact with our healers, and personal involvement in the healing process. Finally, we are distrustful of our own agribusiness and the pharmaceutical industry. Therefore, we look for organic foods to put in our mouths whenever we have a reasonable opportunity. And we pursue practices such as tai chi and yoga to promote our own health.

Nevertheless, when an epidemic emerges, be it caused by ebola virus, HIV, or avian flu, the world looks to Western medicine. The whole idea of complementary medicine is to strengthen, deepen, and widen the application of these and other techniques, using them together. Anesthesia by itself is no cure, surgery without anesthesia may be intolerable, but used together they have saved many lives. Yoga may add usefully to treatments for pain, combining with medicines, massage, physical therapy, acupuncture, or other adjunctive therapies such as Alexander technique to yield a synergy that is very much to the patient's advantage.

Many of the *asana*, or yoga postures, that we offer in this book might look familiar to any of you who have done stretching or calisthenics. In fact, there has been a good deal of interchange in both directions; a fair number of *asana* originating from other types of physical culture such as gymnastics were then described in yoga texts within the last few centuries.[4] At some point, from one source or another, they have been adopted and adapted by body workers. Physiatrists, physical therapists, instructors of Alexander, Feldenkrais, Pilates, and Kinetic Awareness, and other types of therapists may recognize some of the postures and strategies that we are about to describe. One response might be, "I've already seen this. There's nothing new here." Others with the same knowledge base might react, "We already do some of this. We know it is effective. Let's see if there are additional maneuvers, combinations, applications, or refinements that can benefit our patients." It is along the lines of the second attitude that we have written this book.

How one does yoga can make just as much difference as *what* one does. When the body is unbalanced (e.g., a chronically curved spine or a shoulder held too far forward), the muscles, tendons, and ligaments are under constant strain. Weak or contracted muscles fall prey to a vicious cycle of misalignment and asymmetrical strain, which then causes pain and perpetuates disuse. Conversely, good alignment supports optimal functioning, which in many cases will relieve pain. The preparations for the poses, the alignment of the body in the pose, and the actions done while in the pose are every bit as important as its visual shape. The instructions in the book are fairly detailed for this reason.

Another crucial element in the practice of yoga is one's attitude, or intention. Some people may come to yoga to reduce pain, to relieve stress, to improve strength, balance, or flexibility, or to calm and elevate their consciousness. Some who do yoga have a certain radiance, a sense of peace despite the stresses and strains of life. To set an intention helps to infuse the practice with meaning, and ensures a deeper transformation on every level. We recommend that you give this some thought and formulate your own intention for your practice. A look at the history and philosophy of yoga might help you to do that.

Yoga History and Philosophy

Yoga has been passed down from teacher to pupil for thousands of years in a personal way. Yet yoga is still singular and distinctive, easily recognizable in spite of many millions of practitioners who have lived and passed away, all without an overarching regulatory organization. Although there are many branches and approaches to yoga, its principles and practices present an integral whole.

With little or no clergy and many styles, there are historical texts and traditions that delineate what most yogis might consider to be a full yoga practice. Perhaps the best known one is the *Yoga Sutra*, believed to be written near the beginning of the Common Era by a physician, grammarian, and yogi named Patanjali. This text forms the basis of what is known as "Classical Yoga."[5] A later tradition known as Tantra developed in the seventh to ninth century CE, utilizing many of the same practices but with a different slant. Whereas the Classical yogi's aim is to transcend the body, which is seen to be *inferior* to spirit, Tantra sees no duality and honors the body as a manifestation of the highest consciousness. The body and mind are not obstacles to be overcome, but rather a matrix in which spiritual growth unfolds. In this world view, all experiences, however mundane, provide possibilities for a deeper understanding, and appreciation, of life. There is nothing in life that is inherently separate from spirit.

The practices of Hatha Yoga that are prevalent today draw on both the Classical and Tantric traditions. An ever-increasing number of groups promote both aspects of yoga, from the Iyengar Institute and John Friend's Anusara Yoga to the *Yoga Journal*, among others. Most of these organizations have high aims, consistent with the origins of yoga. All, to our knowledge, embrace the lion's share of the principles set out in Patanjali's *Yoga Sutra*.

Patanjali identifies eight stages, or limbs, of yoga practice, the first seven of which are essential for the eighth.

1. *Yama*, ethical principles, having to do with one's relationship to society (all of which have near equivalents in the ten commandments of the Bible):
   > *Ahimsa*, nonviolence (do not harm oneself or others)
   > *Satya*, truthfulness (do not bear false witness)
   > *Asteya*, honesty (do not steal)
   > *Brahmacharya*, moderation in sense pleasures (do not commit adultery, do not be a glutton, etc.)
   > *Aparigraha*, noncovetousness (do not covet)
2. *Niyama*, personal disciplines
   > *Saucha*, purity
   > *Santosa*, contentment (an actual commandment to be satisfied)
   > *Tapas*, effort or discipline
   > *Svadhyaya*, introspection and study
   > *Isvara-pranidhana*, dedication to a supreme being of no particular denomination or, say some Buddhists, to an underlying unity within the universe
3. *Asana*, physical exercises
4. *Pranayama*, breathing exercises
5. *Pratyahara*, withdrawal of the senses
6. *Dharana*, contemplation
7. *Dhyana*, meditation
8. *Samadhi*, absorption in the Absolute

Contained in the first two stages or limbs are attitudes that will help even a beginning yoga student to gain maximum benefit. When practicing *ahimsa*, or nonviolence, the yoga student will take care not to overwork or strain when performing the poses, even through the medium of a book. *Ahimsa* applies to oneself and others equally. Being clear about one's condition and physical limitations, the practice of *satya*, or truth, forms the basis of an intelligent approach to yoga. On the other hand, one can be too cautious, and in that situation, more *tapas*, or effort, is called for. One should practice yoga without grasping for immediate results, *aparigraha*, developing a healthy patience in the process of learning. As awareness develops, one can more easily appreciate life, and one's movement through it, with *santosa,* or contentment. These first two limbs of Classical Yoga, often omitted from class instructions, can make a huge difference in the experience and outcome of yoga practice.

Another fundamental teaching of yoga is *abhyasa*, or constant practice over a long period of time. Patience and perseverance are recognized as essential to successful yoga. We hope that you experience benefits right away, but those benefits will deepen and consolidate over time with consistent and earnest effort.

The third limb, *asana*, or posture, is the main focus of this book. From the physical standpoint, *asana* are a means to acquire sound balance, healthy strength, coordination, full ranges of motion, and deftness in every limb. Many poses have names based on their silhouette, such as Vrksasana (the tree), Bakasana (the crane), and Dhanurasana (the bow). Others are named for the mood they convey, after heroes or gods in Hindu mythology, such as Virabhadrasana (after a historical warrior) and Hanumanasana (after the mythological figure of Hanuman, the monkey god, the epitome of strength and devoted service). Still others are named for outstanding features in their execution, such as Salamba Sirsasana, or headstand. A balanced practice consists of poses that evoke strength, flexibility, focus, and balance in a variety of ways.

A fair and growing number of Western-style studies[6] have shown yoga to have specific, measurable physiological and psychological benefits such as improved stamina,[7] increased grip strength,[8] better range of motion,[9] reduced pain in arthritis,[10] better control of asthma and diabetes,[11] greater versatility in learning new skills,[12] cortical thickening,[13] lower blood pressure and heart rate,[14] decreased anxiety,[15] better walking,[16] improved autonomic functions such as sleep,[17] reduced back pain,[18] and help in late-stage disease.[19] In one historic view, the *asana* help to stabilize the body and mind, rendering the practitioner ready for meditation. In the Tantric view, the *asana* provide a playful and varied way to express the inner spirit inherent in us all, and also to clarify the subtle energy of the body and its pathways to an inner experience.

The next limb is *pranayama*, techniques to bring greater fullness, ease, and subtlety to the process of breathing. The techniques of *pranayama* have been successfully employed to treat asthma, depression,[20] and other respiratory and psychiatric conditions,[21] but *pranayama* is intended to progress students beyond mere health, bringing them toward higher states of spiritual awareness. As the *Hatha Yoga Pradipika* explains, "When the *prana* (breath) and the *manas* (mind) have been absorbed, an indefinable joy ensues."[22]

Pratyahara, the fifth limb, begins with the yogi turning his or her attention inside and withdrawing from the pull of the senses. Seeing, smelling, hearing, feeling, and tasting all draw the yogi outward toward the world of enticements, whereas the discipline of turning inward through pratyahara makes the yogi receptive to inner, more contemplative realms of experience.

Dharana, concentration, comes after the body has been tempered through *asana*, the mind is invigorated through *pranayama*, and the seductive powers of the senses are controlled through *pratyahara*. Essentially, this is concentrating and focusing the mind, the very heart of the matter, "the still point of the turning wheel, where the fire and the rose are one," as Elliot wrote in "The Wasteland."[23] This single-pointedness or ekagrata is essential for the final two stages.

Dhyana, or meditation, is not easy to capture in words, but can best be understood by experience. Some definitions include "a higher form of awareness";[24] "a form of centering, which involves our disengagement from the machine of the mind and our resting in the heart";[25] "coming into relationship with our own consciousness";[26] and "the basis of all inner work . . . which shifts our understanding of who we are and gives us the power to stand firmly in the center of our being."[27] There are many different styles of meditation with varying techniques. What is common to all is the intention to turn our attention inside and discover an untapped reservoir of ineffable understanding, peace, and joy that is within each of us.

The eighth and final limb is *samadhi*, which is translated as enlightenment, ecstasy, absorption, or union. In the Classical view, *samadhi* is achieved when we separates ourselves from the constantly changing world of everyday life in order to reach liberation. The spirit and the body are seen to be necessarily separate. Tantra philosophy promotes a very different idea of how liberation can be reached. This philosophy understands the body and mind to be our vehicle and "operating system" in this life, but not *inferior* to or separate from spirit. Spirit is embodied and expressed as each one of us, and with this understanding, the physical yoga practice becomes an active form of meditation, a celebration of spirit, rather than a mechanical exercise leading to transcendence. The goal of the Tantric Yoga practice is not to disconnect from life, but to fully embrace it as divine. Tantra in the West has been misconstrued to be synonymous with carnality and sexuality, although actually its fundamental principle is that all existence is sacred.

Whereas Hatha Yoga in Patanjali's time consisted primarily of postures for meditation, the wide spectrum of Hatha Yoga poses that we know today are the products of creative interpretation and experimentation over the last few centuries.[28] Teachers and practitioners alike will continue to discover new avenues and methods toward greater freedom, drawing on yoga's rich history while offering new insights, some based on medicine, science, sports, dance, and the other arts. Yoga is not an "ice palace" that has been preserved without response from the living, changing culture in which it is embedded. Yoga has always been an eclectic tradition, morphing as it grows. You are part of this process.

CHAPTER 3

The Physiology of Yoga

Although yoga is not a science, it can be studied. The principles of its function—how it has the effects it does have—can be understood. After all, fishing is not a science but we can investigate why it works and how to improve it, how to make it more effective. In fact, yoga's traditional practice of stretching muscles and joints and remaining in positions for extended periods of time exploits powerful reflexes and produces a number of salutary effects. These nearly universal responses are as good a place as any to begin.

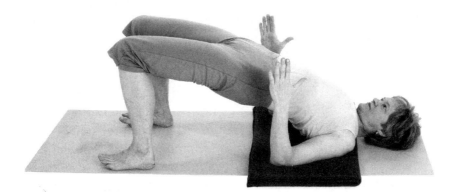

Reflexes

Three common reflexes are used in most of the hundreds of widely practiced yoga poses. The first two reflexes, a system of checks and balances, are almost always a part of yoga. You might have learned about them in high school.

Every muscle in the body has a pair of reflexes that govern its activity. Whenever a muscle is stretched, one reflex—the stretch or myotatic reflex—stimulates the muscle to contract; the other—the Golgi tendon reflex—inhibits muscular contraction in response to stretch. Both reflexes start from tiny sense organs within each muscle and tendon that relay information back to the spinal cord.

When the reflexes that promote or facilitate muscle contraction get triggered, the muscles pull back. They are the ones that respond when the doctor strikes the tendon just below your kneecap. That quick little stretch of the quadriceps muscle results in a tightening of the muscle, contracting it and raising your lower leg. These reflexes are initiated by sense organs, the intrafusal fibers, but these organs also have tiny muscles within them! This allows them to adjust how strongly they stimulate the contraction of large skeletal muscles.

Another set of sense organs in each muscle's tendon—the Golgi tendon organs—inhibit muscle contraction. When there is a tug on a muscle, be it by the hand of a good friend, the swing of a tennis racket, gravity, or yoga, these sense organs contact the spinal and pontine motor centers in the brain to modulate down the tone and actual contraction of every one of the body's muscles.[1]

One basic mechanism in many yoga postures—entering them slowly and holding them—utilizes the fact that the intrafusal (stimulating) fibers are dynamic. Their response is adjustable and proportional to the speed of the stretch. Since they adjust internally to tension, they generally respond less to slow movements and have their greatest influence early in the process of muscle stretching.[2] Their influence fades fast, though, especially if the muscle just stays at its new length.[3] The inhibitory Golgi tendon organs damp down muscle contraction with a force that is weaker than the positive contraction-producing stimulus of the intrafusal fibers. But they continue to exert the same amount of inhibitory influence, at their original strength, over long periods of time.[4] After a while, their

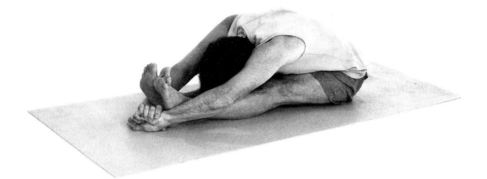

constant input outstrips the diminishing influence of the intrafusal fibers. This naturally tends to reduce a muscle's contractile force as a yoga pose is held.

After a short time—less than two minutes—the muscle will become quiet and stretch more easily and less painfully. Any sustained muscle stretch will eventually bring about a relaxation response in any muscle.[5] Naturally, any painful stimuli that appear during that same time period will have a contrary, unsettling, and excitatory effect.[6] The yoga poses that have lasted over the centuries succeed in accomplishing sustained stretch and relaxation without undue antagonistic, painful, or arousing stimuli.

Speaking of antagonistic, a third reflex is also, albeit very generally, at work during yoga postures. Every skeletal muscle has an antagonist, or direct counterpart: one set of muscles clasps the hand, another opens it. In order for one group of muscles to create a bend at the elbow, the muscles that straighten it must relax. This phenomenon, the agonist-antagonist reflex, is coordinated in the central nervous system and is nearly ubiquitous in Iyengar and Anusara Yoga. If you care to stretch the hamstring muscles, proceed by tightening the quadriceps, and the hamstrings will miraculously relax.[7]

Tightening the quadriceps to straighten the leg at the knee will stretch the hamstring muscles and their golgi tendon organs too, and soon the hamstrings will relax and stretch more and more easily.

Overview

There are several advantages to relaxed and extended muscles in a comfortable and calm individual. In people with arthritis of any type, and really in anyone threatened with decreased range of motion, reducing resistance to motion is an obvious (and painless) means to increase that range. But when arthritis grossly reshapes, distorts, or tightens joints—when just stretching muscles will not do the trick—yoga will render the process of increasing mobility more pleasant and calming, and therefore easier to endure.

However, in the vast majority of joints with restricted motion, where a leathery resistance is felt at the endpoints of movement, the cause is not a deformed joint but constricted joint capsules, tightened ligaments, or muscle shortening. Yoga is the perfect "minimal medicine" in such situations. It is now time to analyze the joints and the most common conditions that come up in arthritis, and then demonstrate the actual remedies that yoga has to offer.

The largest joints in the body are the knees; the smallest are between the bones in the ear. But all moving joints, whether in the wrists, the spine, or the jaw, have the same parts: bones, with cartilage at their interfaces; ligaments that hold them together; and tendons that cross the joints, attaching muscles to the various bones in order to move them when they contract. But there's more to it. All this is described and pictured in Chapter 1.

Osteoarthritis from a Medical Perspective

Osteoarthritis grows from mechanical defects in the surfaces of the joint cartilage and from irregular spawning of new cartilage by the underlying cartilage-making cells.[8] This makes for an uneven distribution of pressures within the joints, and irregular force on the bones beneath the cartilage, which also slowly disrupts the bone substance beneath the joint's cartilage. Subsequently there is further irregularity in the cartilage and yet further distortion of the bone beneath. This process occurs with normal wear and tear in all of us, but our genetic makeup, our activity, and the environment in which we live influence the effects on our joints.

Typically, the cartilage seems to suffer first. In the knee, for example, the normal space between the femur (thigh bone) and the tibia is a centimeter or more. But as time goes on, and at any rate by the mid-fifties, the inner part of most knee joints shows no more than seven or eight millimeters of separation. The medial meniscus, the cartilage that lies on the upper inner surface of the tibia, has begun to thin. Does this happen because the cells making cartilage, the chondrocytes, have slowed down? Or is there some intrinsic change in the quality of the collagen that the cells are producing? Is it just that pressures have, over the years, simply compressed all of the healthy elements together so that they take up less space? Does the underlying bone change on its own? Or are there individually unrecognizable traumas that cumulatively mount to destroy the original arrangement of blood vessels, the subsequent order of the chondrocytes in the cartilage itself, and the matrix of collagen and background fluids until they are no longer adapting to and cushioning the movements of the joint? Do age, strength, activity, hormones, nutrition, exposure to the sun, or even attitude figure into it?

The answer to all these questions is yes, but it is a qualified yes: Different genetic combinations and body types make some factors more important in one individual than in another, and variations in some of the factors change the impact of others. For example, if you do not have enough protein in your system, no amount of exercise will nourish the cartilage sufficiently. If you are hyperthyroid, your cartilage will grow beyond its normal confines. But a good deal of low-impact joint movement is bound to improve circulation and range of motion, almost no matter what.[9]

How Does Osteoarthritis Progress?

Cartilage has a unique type of collagen called type II collagen. It is made of a long, thin string of proteins (proteoglycans) with complex side-chain glycosaminoglycans attached. The arrangement resembles a bottle-washing brush, with a protein at the center and the glycosaminoglycans acting as bristles.

The glycosaminoglycans have negative charges which attract water molecules between them. When there is pressure on the joint, and consequently on the cartilage, the water molecules are reluctantly released, cushioning the pressure and giving a wonderful resilience to the cartilage.[10] Changes in the molecular structure of the proteoglycans are thought to be the basic force in osteoarthritis.[11] These changes acceler-

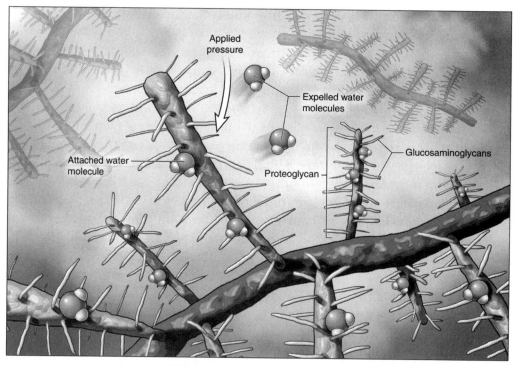

Type II Collagen in Cartilage Matrix under Pressure

Figure 4. Proteins attract the water molecules between their side branches. The water resists as it is squeezed out under pressure. Once the pressure ends, the water returns, the proteins stiffen and expand again. The entire process makes the cartilage elastic and protects the joint.

ate the process of degeneration and impede repair at the surfaces of cartilage, and they might be involved in the unusual and restricting boney formations and ligamentous damage that are so often seen in degenerative arthritis throughout the body.[12]

Adult chondrocytes no longer multiply, but they do respond to damage, "eating" the degenerated cartilage and using the molecular building blocks to create new, healthy strands of it. The enzymes that help digest the old cartilage are more abundant where osteoarthritis is present.[13] Metabolism in general is up. The processes of degeneration and repair are going on simultaneously, but over time the repair cannot keep up with the degeneration. Less elastic forms of cartilage appear, which increases the stresses on the bone below, causing microfractures. After the microfractures heal, the bone is less supple and less elastic. This concentrates the shock waves of pressure inherent in so many forms of action, focuses them on the cartilage, and promotes even more degeneration.

This process also produces sufficiently great pressures on the bones that they react, as bones must, by laying down new bone substance in the areas of greatest stress. The production of osteophytes may be the response of bone to the eccentric stresses brought about by the degenerative process. Unfortunately, just as the cartilage is getting thin, the underlying bone is changing shape, altering still further the patterns of stress for which the joint was originally so well adapted.

There is more to learn about osteoarthritis. It was recently shown that brief stimulation "winds up" neurons inside the joint and at the spinal cord and brain, making them more reactive to future stimuli. In addition, peripheral and central sensitization, in effect, make a person feel greater pain from the same cause.[14] Further, the stimulated pain fibers in the joint actually give off substances that attack cartilage.[15] Like eddies in a rushing stream, in arthritis one vicious cycle leads to others. These silent destructive forces may have an equally silent and equally effective antidote.

There is good reason to believe that the calming effect of yoga is beneficial here. Soothing, relaxing physical activity is beneficial after cardiac events and in people with asthma or hypertension. Where hyperexcitability of the nervous system is part of the problem, yoga has often been part of the solution. But this has yet to be demonstrated empirically. Verifying the efficacy of practical yoga solutions to medical problems is now a reality.[16] Sometimes significant advances are made by practitioners like you.

But to become a practitioner, one must practice. In the next chapter we offer you some guidance based on our experience that will make yoga safer, maximally effective, and more fun.

CHAPTER 4

Prelude to the Poses

Integrative Medicine

Historically, yoga coexisted with Ayurvedic medicine, nutritional remedies, astrologers, snake charmers, shamans, and various religious means to cure illness. Today we have a similar array of sciences and healing modalities that can be used concurrently. It does a patient no good to ignore, either from choice or from ignorance, other means of healing. At times, using two methods concurrently is much better than either attempted alone. We must resist Classical Yoga's tendency toward

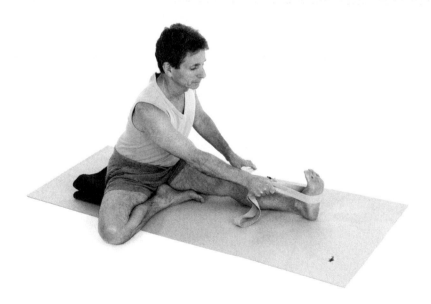

independence and purity for the good of the person with arthritis. Later, some practitioners will be able to proceed with yoga alone, and leave behind the scaffolding that helped them to that fortunate point.

Yoga off the Mat

As your body awareness improves through this practice, you will be able to adjust your postural and movement patterns in a more refined way while involved in your normal daily activities. You will recognize opportunities to let yoga inform your movements and posture for the better.

The Poses

The poses we have chosen are a combination of classical *asana* and variations or excerpts of poses that have particular therapeutic benefit. The poses in each chapter are arranged to be practiced in sequence, which has its own logic, but once you have tried to do all the poses, you should concentrate most on the ones that feel right to you. Poses with *stages* have progressive levels of difficulty; the *variations* to poses give alternatives requiring equal skill.

The Chapters

We begin with ubiquitous poses. They appear so frequently throughout what follows that they deserve a chapter of their own, which we call "The All-Stars." Look at them while you are fresh; done properly, there is something wonderful about each one. The All-Star poses can be done as a complete practice by those wanting a general arthritis-preventing regime. After the All-Star chapter, each subsequent chapter is specific to a joint or a condition. We describe each joint before going into the poses. It helps to understand what is going on inside your body, and how you might work around your physical difficulties in daily life. Education is preferable to medication. You cannot overdose on education. It does not expire. The main side effect is curiosity. But be careful, knowledge is addictive: after a certain amount of exposure, you want more and more.

Where an All-Star pose appears in a later chapter on a specific joint, it is identified by an asterisk and an identifying picture stands

alongside the name. We suggest that you refer to the full description of
the pose in the All-Star chapter on the page cited. You may also want to
practice a version of the pose that is different from the one pictured.
For instance, Adho Mukha Svanasana is listed in the chapter on shoulders, and you may choose to do the variation with a wall (Wall Dog)
instead of the full pose. If the variation is sufficiently different from
the All-Star, then there will be neither an asterisk nor a small picture,
but rather the pose will have a full description with illustrative pictures
just like any other pose. If the departure from the All-Star is slight,
then you will see the asterisk, the small picture, and an instruction
describing the change.

Other poses also have variations. At times we refer to the basic
pose, and number the variations' instructions by just continuing the
numbering of the basic pose. At other times we start over with new
instructions, pictures, and numbers. The decision depends on just how
different the variation is.

At the end of each chapter is a table indicating which poses address
which ranges of motion for that joint. The tables are not uniform. They
are designed to help readers and therapists efficiently design programs
that focus on one or several joints or problems. There is no table in the
chapter on scoliosis, since all of the poses there are aimed at correcting
spinal curves.

Contraindications

Contraindications, or reasons for not attempting a pose, are of two
types. One type is *absolute*. If you have an absolute contraindication, do
not do that pose. The second type is *relative*, which means you should
use extreme caution and vigilance when you attempt the pose, but with
sufficient care the pose might be done. These poses are often best initiated with a teacher or therapist. All contraindications are relative unless
stated as absolute.

Of course we cannot mention every possible contraindication to
any pose. However, we can categorically discourage doing yoga less
than three to five hours after a full meal. The best general advice we
can give about yoga and arthritis in just about any context is to use common sense.

Working from a Book

Reading this book while you are doing the poses may prove to be cumbersome, so you can try different approaches: Read the instructions through several times and "rehearse" the pose in your mind, then do it without the book in your hands. Or have a friend or teacher or physical therapist read the instructions out loud while you do the poses. You might also tape-record them. With repetition you will remember the most important elements, and then you can review the instructions periodically to see if you have missed anything. Please be sure to read all the instructions for each pose before attempting it; do not skip over the preparations. These details about placement and actions will greatly increase the effectiveness, safety, and enjoyment of your practice.

Props

In addition to the yoga mat, we suggest the use of props such as chairs, blocks, blankets, or straps. These can ease you into poses that would otherwise be dangerous or impossible. For example, a man with a colostomy may not be able to lie on his stomach directly, but with two or three folded blankets placed under the chest and under the pelvis, it would be easy. If your legs are tight and you are reaching for the floor, shortening your reach by use of a block is sensible.

A Word about Words

There is something we have noticed about teaching yoga that is a perpetual source of wonder: people, entire yoga classes, respond to directions that in themselves might not make much sense. Mr. Iyengar has often said, "Make space in your lower back" or "Relax your ears." Yet people hear these obscure commands, and they all do the same thing, which is exactly what is intended. Please be tolerant in what you read. Rather than analyzing each direction, let it direct you. You, and your yoga, will be better for it.

The instructions offered here are inspired by both Iyengar Yoga and Anusara Yoga, developed by John Friend. Mr. Iyengar created many,

many beautiful poses and developed others in a way that combines classical knowledge with solid physiological instinct, geometrical precision, and hard work—especially the hard work. John Friend, who studied extensively with Mr. Iyengar, worked with these well-wrought *asana*, and formulated principles based on everything he had learned. Friend's methods lend themselves well to teaching beginners by promoting awareness, alignment, and enthusiasm in a user-friendly way. Throughout the text we express many universal concepts through the methods of Anusara Yoga. Mr. Iyengar's teachings are implicit in the instructions and are also guiding us throughout. If you want to study either or both of these methods more deeply, you will need a teacher. See the Resources section for details.

The word *firm* is usually encountered as a noun, as in a law firm, or an adjective, as in the request "Be firm with him." Here we use it as a verb: "Firm the muscles of your thigh," meaning contract or tighten them, but with care. We use *tone* as a synonym for *firm*. We also use *root* as a verb to mean reach down into the foundation of the pose as roots of a tree reach into the earth.

Medical words, especially as they appear in the contraindications section, might be unfamiliar. We have tried to anticipate this and defined them in the glossary.

Your Attitude

Each pose requires focus and a willing intellect and body. One of the best practitioners we know approached yoga originally (at age four) as a form of play. Although the purpose is absolutely serious, that may be the right attitude. There is a tradition for this in Indian lore. In the midst of rival armies arrayed before the great battle set forth in the *Mahabharata*, Arjuna asks Krishna why the universe was created. Krishna smilingly replies, "For sport." Some of the most serious things are best done in dedicated high spirits.

Respect your body and listen to its signals, including the pleasure and comfort of stretching in the poses, and pain and fatigue. Learn to distinguish between the discomfort of stretching a tight muscle or joint and the pain of overstretching. In the same way, learn to identify the heaviness of lethargy that will dissipate as you move, as opposed to true fatigue that tells you to stop and rest.

How to Begin and Finish

We often show you the full classical pose even though sometimes you might not be able to do it right away. In any event, just seeing it will give you the Gestalt, an idea of what you are aiming for, what you are starting out to do.

Set the foundation, the part of you that touches the floor, carefully, and be aware of the details. To prepare for a pose, breathe in. Breathe out as you go into the pose, and breathe normally while holding the pose. Decide for yourself how long to hold the pose, and do not obsess about timing; your body will tell you. You can use a timer or your intuitive clock. Do not count. To finish the pose, inhale and return to the position in which you began the pose while still active in the body. Do not let go of your focus or your energy until you have come out of the pose fully. Finally, take the time after each pose to feel its effects. At the end of any practice session, rest in a comfortable sitting or lying position for five to ten minutes. Let the effects of practice settle in.

CHAPTER 5

The All-Stars

We start with a group of poses that are helpful for a number of joints. They reappear in each of the later chapters. Taken together, these All-Stars make up an excellent assortment of *asana* for people who have mild generalized arthritis or who want to avoid acquiring any significant joint limitations in the future. For those who would like a Sanskrit name for this group, we can suggest Mukhya Artha (Primary Purpose) or Sarva Artha (All Purpose).

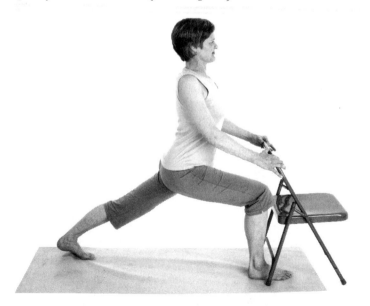

1. TADASANA (Mountain Pose)

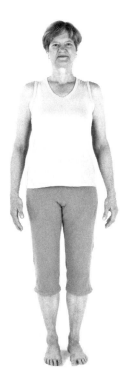

Purpose: To establish well-aligned posture and *stillness* that will apply to all standing poses.

Contraindications: Severe imbalance, plantar fasciitis.

Props: None.

Avoiding pitfalls: Because one's posture is habitual, extra care is needed to refine this most basic standing pose. Use a mirror to observe your alignment from the side and front. Common errors: pushing the pelvis too far forward, flattening the lower back, slumping the chest. Try to maintain a vertical plumb line through your whole body, from ankles to knees to hips to shoulders to ears. Respect the natural curves of the spine.

INSTRUCTIONS:

1. Stand with your feet hip-width apart and parallel, legs straight, arms hanging at your sides.
2. Balance the weight as evenly as you can between the four corners of your feet (see page 235): the inner heel, the mound of the big toe, the little toe mound, and the outer heel.
3. Lift the inner arches by raising your toes, then retain the arch lift as you lower your toes.
4. Take a breath to enliven your body.
5. Firm your leg muscles and bring the tops of your thighs back until they are over your ankles. You are pushing your hips back behind you, but actually this does not distort your posture.
6. Widen your hips and thighs by abducting them away from each other without changing your feet or lower legs.
7. Keep your thighs back and your pelvis wide, then curl your tailbone down to lengthen your spine.
8. Firm and lift your lower abdominal muscles.
9. Stretch upward from your pelvis through your torso and neck, so that your whole spine is long. If your lower back feels too arched, pull back through the sides of your waist.
10. Use the muscles between your shoulder blades to gently draw your shoulders back.

11. Balance your head lightly over the top of your spine. Look straight ahead. Let your arms hang by your sides. Be fully present in all parts of your body; create both a solid foundation and an upward expansion. Embody the dignity of the mountain this pose is named for. How long you hold the pose is up to you.

VARIATIONS:

TADASANA URDHVA HASTASANA
(Mountain Pose with arms reaching up)

1. Inhale and lift your arms out to the side and up to your ears. Make a sweeping movement that stretches your ribs and sides. As you move, the tops of the arms stay close in to the shoulder joints, but the hands and forearms reach out.
2. Exhale as you lower the arms back to your sides.
3. Repeat this several times, following the natural rhythm of your breath.

TADASANA URDHVA BADDHA HASTASANA
(arms up, hands clasped)

1. Repeat the sweeping movement as above to raise your arms.
2. Interlace your fingers and turn the palms up.
3. Extend *strongly* and equally down into the earth and up to the sky.
4. Set the humeri firmly into the shoulder sockets and the elbows as straight as possible.
5. Breathe easily and fully.

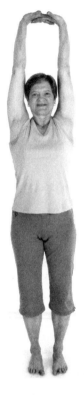

This pose provides a full stretch of the shoulders, arms, and hands.

---

2. STANDING LUNGE WITH WALL

Purpose: To learn pelvic and leg alignment and stretch Achilles tendons and plantar fasciae; to extend and flex the hips and knees.

Contraindications: Achilles tendonitis or bursitis, torn meniscus, plantar fasciitis or anterior cruciate ligment.

Props: A yoga mat and wall.

Avoiding pitfalls: Make sure the pelvis stays square to the wall, the feet parallel, the forward knee over the ankle, and the back thigh lifted away from the floor. Bear your weight equally over the four corners of the feet and lift the arches.

INSTRUCTIONS:

1. Stand facing a wall and place your hands on the wall at a comfortable height, elbows bent.
2. Step the left foot back, keeping both feet and your pelvis facing directly toward the wall.
3. Bend the forward right knee over the ankle. The back heel will be up off the floor.
4. Roll your upper arms and shoulders back.
5. Take a deep breath as you lift your spine up and firm the leg muscles.
6. Lean slightly toward the wall and widen your upper thighs and buttocks apart.
7. Curl the back of the pelvis down and the front part up, drawing your belly in and up.
8. Firmly anchor in your pelvis, bring your shoulders and head back directly over your hips, and shift more weight onto the back foot to lower the heel toward the floor. Hold the back thigh lifted away from the floor.
9. Maintain a balance of strength and expansion.

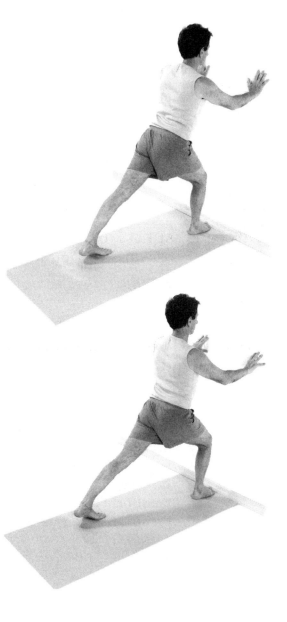

10. To intensify: Place the toes of the front foot up the wall.

11. Step your left foot as far back as you can while maintaining your hips facing squarely toward the wall.

12. Isometrically pull your hands down the wall (without moving them) to lift your chest. Look up.

13. If you feel steady enough, lift your arms up alongside your head as in Tadasana Urdhva Hastasana. Reach up vigorously!

14. Exhale and return to Tadasana, then repeat on the other side.

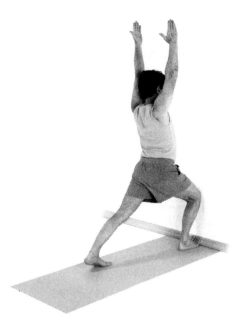

The iliopsoas muscle, a deep hip flexor, often contributes to lumbar stiffness. This pose stretches it.

3. ADHO MUKHA SVANASANA SERIES (Downward Dog in four stages)

Purpose: To extend the spine and stretch the chest and hamstring muscles. The partial inversion in the full pose also strengthens the arms and thoracic spine.

Contraindications: Acromioclavicular dysfunction, rotator cuff tear, thoracic outlet syndrome, spondylolisthesis, severe osteoporosis, carpal tunnel syndrome, Dupuytren's contracture.

Props: A yoga mat, blanket, wall, and tabletop.

Avoiding pitfalls: Retract the shoulder blades firmly onto the back ribs; do not let the upper arms sag downward. Roll the biceps upward to maintain outward rotation of the upper arms. Balance the hands and feet on their four corners. Keep the knees bent if you are stiff, in order to be able to tip the pelvis so the spine can lengthen.

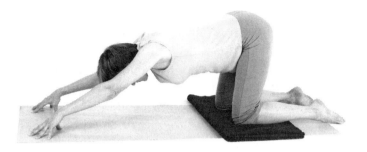

INSTRUCTIONS FOR FOUR STAGES OF THE POSE:

Stage I: Puppy

1. Kneel on a blanket with your shins hip-width apart.
2. Walk your hands forward far enough so that your spine and arms stretch forward at a diagonal. Your hips remain over your knees, your head between your arms.
3. Lift onto your fingertips as shown. This helps to keep your arm muscles active.
4. Arch your sitting bones back and up and apart.
5. Firm your belly and extend forward through your spine and arms.
6. Adjust your upper arms well back and into the shoulder joints.
7. Lift your upper arms with elbows straight.
8. Breathe and soften on the inside as you continue reaching forward with your arms.
9. Walk your hands back to come out of the pose.

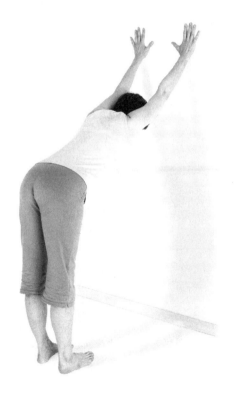

Stage II: Wall Dog

1. Place your hands on the wall above eye level, with your index fingers pointing up and your arms shoulder-width apart.

2. Place your feet hip-width apart and parallel.

3. Straighten your arms and move your chest a little toward the wall.

4. Move your upper arms more securely back into the shoulder joints.

5. Keep your elbows straight and your upper arms light but active.

6. Bend forward through your trunk until there is one long diagonal line from hands to hips. You can step back as needed.

7. Elevate your sitting bones and separate them, which will make an arch in your lower back.

8. Draw in your belly and lengthen the tailbone back.

9. Let the thoracic spine soften downward without your arms collapsing.

10. If your hamstring muscles allow, do the pose with straight legs. If your hamstrings are tight, your knees can bend slightly to allow the pelvis to tilt properly. Find the degree of effort in extending yourself that feels good, using your breath.

11. After several breaths, come back up as you inhale, and step toward the wall.

Stage III: Table Dog

1. Place your hands shoulder-width apart on a tabletop, with your index fingers pointing forward.

2. Tighten the muscles of your arms and secure your arms into the shoulder joints as you gently lower your chest.

3. Inhale, become light inside your torso.

4. Step back enough to fully extend your arms and bend forward with your entire trunk, bending your knees slightly to ensure that you can lengthen your spine. Stretch your arms fully.

5. Arch your sitting bones upward and separate them.

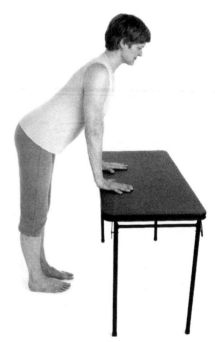

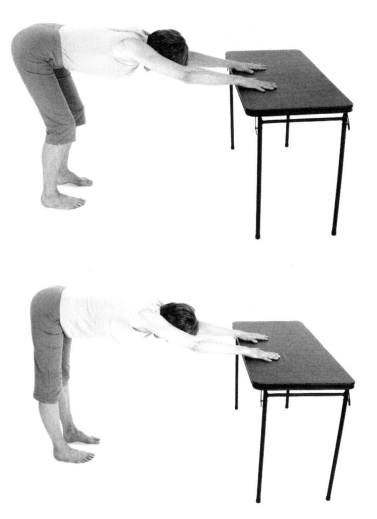

6. Lengthen the tailbone back and firm your lower belly.
7. Lower your upper chest toward the floor without dropping your arms.
8. Stretch fully from your core out through your arms, legs, and spine. If you can, straighten your legs.
9. To come out of the pose, step toward the table and return to Tadasana.

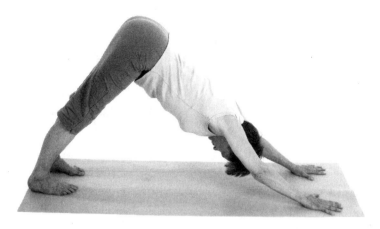

Stage IV: Adho Mukha Svanasana (Full Downward Dog)

1. Come down onto your hands and knees on the mat. Walk your knees back a bit farther than your hips. Place your hands at the front of the mat, shoulder-width apart, with your fingers separated and the index fingers pointing forward.
2. Firm your arm muscles, press your fingers down, and soften your chest down over the tops of the arms so that the upper arms connect solidly into the shoulder sockets.
3. Secure your shoulder blades in toward your spine.
4. Raise your heels, putting the plantar surface of your toes on the mat, and make space in the sides and front of your entire torso.
5. Inhale, lift up your knees and hips, elevating the sitting bones back, up, and apart.
6. As you exhale, extend your arms and spine, pulling your legs back still farther. If your hamstring muscles are very tight, bend your knees to allow your pelvis to tilt properly, and gradually work to straighten your knees.
7. Create a slight concavity in the lumbar and thoracic spine by reaching upward with the sitting bones.
8. As you become more flexible, you will be able to pull the thighs back with straight knees, and eventually lower your heels.
9. Once you have created the full pose, extend with sensitivity through all parts of the body, from the core to the periphery. Charge the body with your intention to open and stretch.
10. To release, bring your knees to the floor.

4. UTTHITA PARSVAKONASANA
(Side Angle Standing Pose)

Purpose: To strengthen and stretch the hips, legs, and spine.

Contraindications: Imbalance, plantar fasciitis, anterior cruciate tear, patellofemoral arthralgia, Dupuytren's contracture.

Props: A yoga mat, a wall, and a block.

Avoiding pitfalls: The back leg may collapse, the front knee may misalign. Use a block for the hand that goes to the floor if your hips are stiff.

INSTRUCTIONS:

1. Stand with your back to a wall, raise your arms to shoulder height, and step your feet apart the same width as your outstretched arms.
2. Turn the right foot and leg parallel to the wall but do not turn the torso.
3. Inhale, firm your legs and lengthen up through the spine. As you exhale, bend your right knee until it is over the ankle. Point the knee toward the second toe.

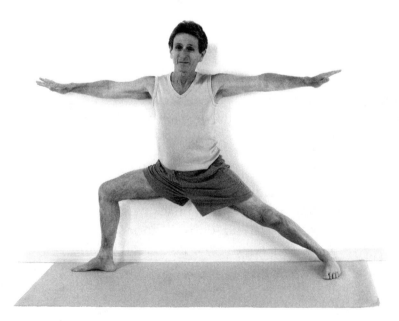

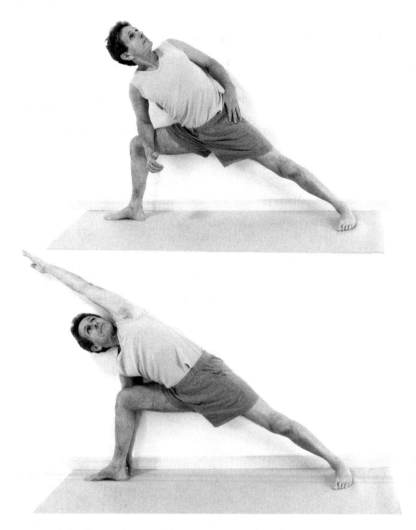

4. As you inhale again, incline your torso over your right hip and rest your right forearm on your thigh. Your left hand rests on your hip.
5. Stabilize the right leg in this position.
6. Anchor the left foot. Move your left thigh back toward the wall, revolving the entire thigh slightly inward at first, toward the midline.
7. Curl your tailbone toward the left heel, tighten your lower belly, and now rotate your left knee outward to face away from the floor. These actions will increase your power and stability.
8. From the pelvis, at the center of the pose, stretch in all directions, pulling your shoulders back toward the wall. Revolve your head to look up.

TO INTENSIFY:

9. Place your right fingertips or palm on the floor or on a block between your right foot and the wall. Extend your left arm up alongside your left ear, as in Tadasana Urdhva Hastasana, continuing the diagonal line of your left leg.

10. Notice the balance of strength and expansion in this exhilarating pose.

11. Inhale as you come back up. Repeat on the other side. You can stand in Tadasana before you repeat the pose on the other side if you wish, to rest and feel the effects.

5. UTTHITA TRIKONASANA (Triangle Pose)

Purpose: To strengthen and stretch the legs, hips, and spine.

Contraindications: Imbalance, pubic fracture.

Props: A yoga mat, a wall, and a block.

Avoiding pitfalls: The wider your stance, the more freedom you will have in the hips, but do not go so wide as to lose stability. The knees may want to bend and the upper body tends to shift

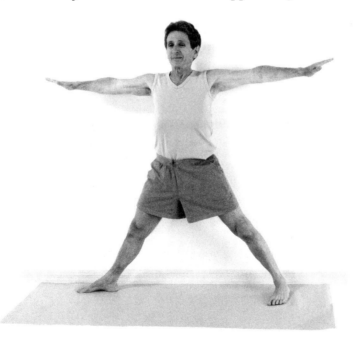

forward. Keep your legs straight, and your torso lined up directly above your legs and parallel to the wall behind you.

INSTRUCTIONS:

1. Stand with your back to the wall, raise your arms to shoulder height, and step your feet apart the same width as your outstretched arms. Turn the right foot and leg parallel to the wall, but face your torso straight out from the wall. Internally rotate the left foot thirty degrees toward the right.

2. With your arms remaining outstretched, incline your torso to the right without bending it. Your hips will shift to the left.

3. Inhale, firm your legs to keep them straight, and lengthen out through the spine. Exhale and shift your hips more to the left. Extend your torso out over your right leg, bending at the hips, not the waist.

4. Distribute your weight more or less equally on both feet.

5. Keep both sides of the torso long and parallel. Avoid collapsing down, but extend the spine horizontally as you widen your thighs. Curl your tailbone down and lift your belly in and up.

6. Place your right hand down on your ankle or on a block.

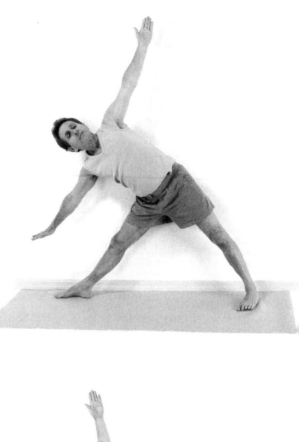

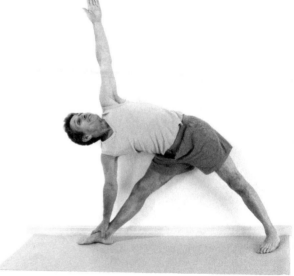

Stretch the left arm straight up. If you are unsteady, lean your hip and one or both shoulders lightly against the wall.

7. Roll your left shoulder, left ribs, and left waist back and up, remaining steady in your legs. Gaze up at your left thumb.

8. Radiate energy out through all your limbs and your spine. Stretch side to side as well as head to tail.

9. Inhale and come back up, with your arms still outstretched.

10. Repeat on the other side. You can stand in Tadasana before repeating the pose on the other side if you wish. This pose builds stamina and focus, as well as stretching the hips and legs.

---

6. PRASARITA PADOTTANASANA (Wide Leg Standing Forward Bend)

Purpose: To stretch the adductors, hamstring muscles, gluteus maximus, and spine, and invert the upper body. This wide-open standing pose helps to develop stamina and self-assurance.

Contraindications: Imbalance, ankle sprain.

Props: A yoga mat and two blocks.

Avoiding pitfalls: Balance the weight on the four corners of the feet; avoid tipping your hips back. Breathe with ease and fullness. Even when the arms are hanging down, pull them up into the shoulder sockets.

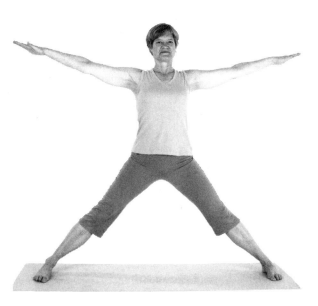

INSTRUCTIONS:

1. Extend your arms out to the sides at shoulder height. Step your feet apart to the width of both outstretched arms. Make sure the feet are parallel. Press the four corners of each foot down, but lift your arches.

2. Inhale, firm your legs, and stretch up through the spine. Exhale, bend forward, retaining the long spine,

and reach straight down to touch the floor or two blocks. You may bend your knees if the hamstring muscles are very tight. It is important to tip the pelvis forward from your hips, not by rounding your waist.

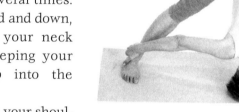

3. Once your hands are on the floor or the blocks, inhale, extend your legs and sitting bones back, and draw your spine forward. Exhale and release your spine and neck. Repeat this breathing/extending movement several times. Then hang forward and down, totally releasing your neck and head but keeping your arms pulled up into the shoulder sockets.

4. To intensify: Move your shoulder blades in toward the spine and toward your lower back. Take hold of both ankles and pull your entire torso farther down. Breathe as you stretch your back fully.

5. To come out of the pose, step your feet a bit closer to each other, bring your hands to your hips, then inhale and stretch your head and chest forward to come up strongly, retracting your shoulder blades as you do so.

6. Step your feet together into Tadasana.

7. STANDING LUNGE WITH CHAIR
(Virabhadrasana variation)

Purpose: To extend the hip, strengthen the quadriceps, stretch the *iliopsoas, pectoralis, latissimus dorsi,* and *teres major* muscles, and promote balance.

Contraindications: Hyperlordosis, spondylolisthesis, spondylolysis, severe lumbar stenosis.

Props: A yoga mat and a chair.

Avoiding pitfalls: Set the pelvis carefully, squarely facing the back of the chair, and keep it that way as you perform the pose. Do not let the back leg droop. Align the front knee with the second toe.

INSTRUCTIONS:

1. Stand facing the back of your chair.
2. Bend the right knee as you step the left foot back. Movement stops when the right shin is vertical.
3. Attentively find the balance between the four corners of the right foot, and the two front corners of the left foot.
4. Lean forward a bit toward the chair, fully stretch your back leg, and firm the muscles from foot to hip.
5. Retain the forward lean, widen the upper thighs and pelvic bones, then lengthen your tailbone down and draw the lower belly in and up to stabilize your pelvis.
6. Bring your torso upright and retract your shoulders back until they are just above your hips.
7. Let go of the chair when ready, and stretch your arms up near your ears. Breathe fully and confidently as you maintain this pose.

---

8. PRESSURE COOKER
(Utkatasana variation)

Purpose: To strengthen thigh abductors and shoulder adductors,

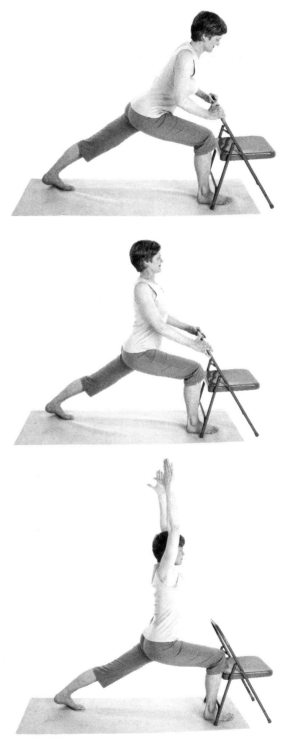

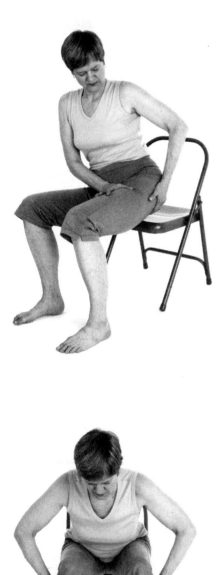

and widen the thighs and pelvis without widening the lower legs. To repair and maintain the hip joints.

Contraindications: Severe hypertension, colostomy, hemorrhoids.

Props: A chair and a belt.

Avoiding pitfalls: Take care in the placement of your legs. Press into the sides of the upper shins firmly enough with your hands to balance the strong outward push with your thighs. *Keep breathing!*

INSTRUCTIONS (TWO VARIATIONS):

Seated variation

1. Sit on a firm chair with your legs parallel and hip-width apart.
2. With both hands on one hip and thigh, manually turn the thigh in and broaden the hip to the side.
3. Perform the same action on the other side as well. This adjustment sets your foundation and allows for the actions that follow to be most effective. In Anusara Yoga this is called "Manual Inner Spiral." See Appendix III for more information about the Inner Spiral.
4. Lean forward and place your hands on the outside of the legs just below your knees. If you have shoulder or arm pain, place a belt to encircle your legs just below the knees instead of using your arms.
5. Widen and retract your sitting bones. Lean forward from your hips, not your waist. Firm all your thigh muscles and inhale as you lengthen out through your spine.
6. As you exhale, push your hands strongly in toward the midline, and press out equally strongly with

your thighs. The resisted isometric movement will widen your pelvis, relieving compression in the hips and sacroiliac joints.

Once you are familiar with this action, you can apply it to many poses even without the actual opposing forces.

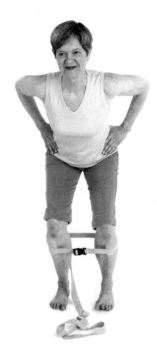

Standing variation

1. Place the belt around your upper shins to maintain alignment of the lower legs.
2. Bend your knees and lean forward slightly, hands on your hips.
3. Strongly widen your thighs, from the hips to the knees, and breathe, keeping your spine long.
4. After several deep breaths, release the action and stand back up.

This pose offers a good opportunity to practice intense effort without holding your breath or becoming agitated. Trust the process of building strength and awareness.

---

9. CHAIR TWIST (Bharadvajasana variation)

Purpose: To rotate the spine, mobilize its joints, and learn how to stabilize the pelvis while twisting.

Contraindications: Herniated cervical or lumbar nucleus pulposus, spondylolisthesis, spondylolysis, total hip replacement.

Prop: A chair.

Avoiding pitfalls: Avoid overworking the arms and neck to achieve the twist. Keep the pelvis and legs stable and aligned as instructed.

INSTRUCTIONS:

1. Sit sideways in a firm chair without arms, with your right side close to the chair back. Set your legs hip-width apart and parallel, with your knees vertically over your ankles.

2. Firm your leg muscles, manually widen your buttocks and upper thighs as in Pressure Cooker above, then sit tall with awareness of your spine as your central core.

3. Reach your tailbone lightly downward and lift your lower belly to lengthen and stabilize the lower spine.

4. Inhale, lengthen through your whole torso, and retract your shoulder blades together behind you so that the actions of your arms will affect your torso and spine.

5. Exhale, turn to the right, and take hold of the chair in a way that helps you turn more deeply.

6. Coordinate your actions with your breath, inhaling as you lengthen your spine and exhaling as you turn farther. Use the rhythm of your breath to coax more movement through your body.

7. To keep your hips and pelvis aligned, pull your left thigh back into the hip socket. This will counteract the normal tendency for the pelvis to turn with the spine. The more strongly you use your arms, the more important it is to retract the shoulders and upper arms to distribute the force of the twist.

8. Return to the center. Prepare to twist to the left by turning to the other side of the chair.

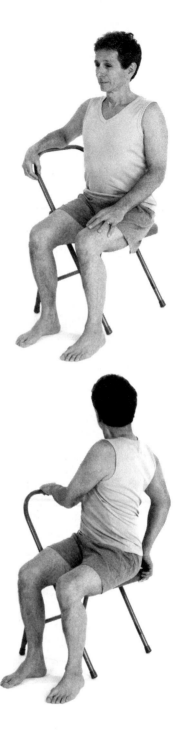

10. WALL QUAD (Eka Pada Rajakapotasana variation)

Purpose: To extend the hip and stretch all four of the quadriceps one leg at a time.

Contraindications: Prepatellar bursitis, knee effusion, hyperlordosis.

Props: A chair, one or two folded blankets, and a pad.

Avoiding pitfalls: Keep the pelvis squared to the direction you are facing, do not let one hip go back or forward. Line up each leg from hip to knee to ankle.

INSTRUCTIONS:

1. Place the back of a chair against a wall, and a folded blanket on the floor beside it. If you have a pad, put it along the wall. Sit on the front left corner of your chair and manually broaden your thighs and hips, as in the Pressure Cooker.

2. Step your right foot forward on the floor until it is under your bent knee and facing straight forward. Bend the left knee, rest it on the folded blanket, and raise your foot up the wall. Use more padding under your knee as needed. Try to align the thigh vertically, with the knee directly under or behind the hip.

3. Firm the muscles of both legs, and widen your sitting bones and upper thighs.

4. Lengthen your tailbone down and pull your belly in and up. The stretch will be more intense the closer your knee is to the wall, and the more you pull the tailbone down.

5. Breathe, and stretch up through your spine as well. Be patient! This stretch will pay off over time.

6. Lean to the right side to free the left leg and change sides.

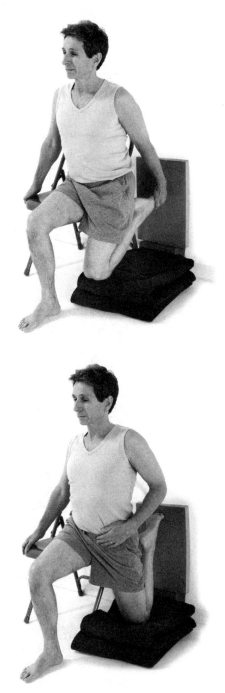

11. LOTUS PREP WITH WALL
(Ankle-to-Knee Lotus Preparation)

Purpose: To stretch the hip and outer thigh (iliotibial band), expanding range of motion in a position that keeps the spine elongated.

Contraindications: Cerebrovascular disease, severe hypertension, colostomy, gastric reflux, medial meniscal tear, lateral collateral ligamentous sprain, severe joint effusion.

Props: A yoga mat and a wall, a blanket under your head for comfort if needed.

Avoiding pitfalls: Hold the pelvis flat on the floor and evenly placed left to right. Keep the foot of your crossover leg flexed to protect your knee. You may find that you are tighter on one side than the other; move farther away from the wall when crossing over with the tighter side.

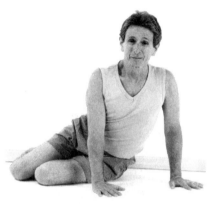

INSTRUCTIONS:

1. Sit on the floor parallel to a wall. The closer you are to the wall, the more challenging the pose. Start with your

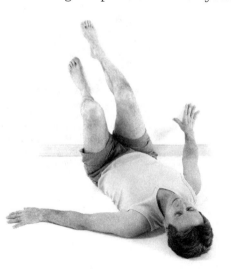

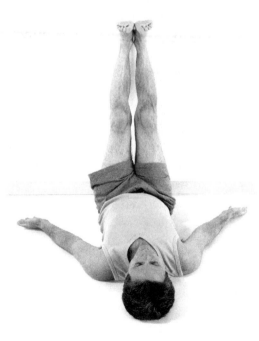

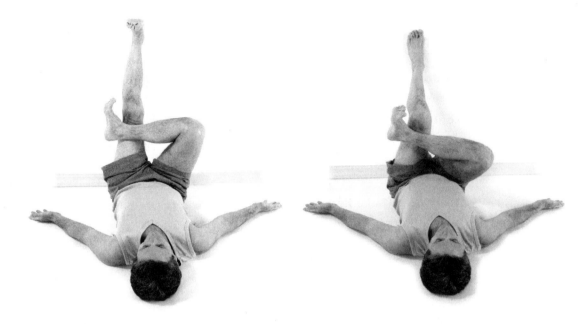

hips about twelve inches away from the wall and move closer to the wall later as it becomes feasible.

2. "Walk up" the wall as you move your torso out from it until your feet are up the wall, and your torso is perpendicular to it. You may have a blanket under your head if you wish.

3. Cross your right foot over the left knee and flex your right ankle, pulling the toes, especially the fourth and fifth toes, straight back toward your knee.

4. Take a breath, expand yourself inside, and curl your sitting bones down, which will arch your lower back away from the floor.

5. Slide your left foot down the wall. Keep going until you can no longer maintain the square and flat-to-the-floor alignment of your pelvis.

6. Stay in this position. Continue to pull your sitting bones down and apart.

7. Firm your lower abdomen and stretch out through your spine. Patiently give the hip and thigh time to stretch.

8. To release and change sides, slide the left foot back up the wall.

12. WINDSHIELD WIPER (distant relative of Jathara Parivartanasana)

Purpose: To internally rotate the hips, one at a time, to stretch the side of the body, and to encourage full relaxed breathing.

Contraindications: Total hip replacement (prosthetic hip should not overly adduct), colostomy, herniated lumbar disc.

Props: A yoga mat, possibly a blanket under your head for comfort.

Avoiding pitfalls: Be sure to start with your legs wide apart, and adjust the position of your arms for comfort.

INSTRUCTIONS:

1. Lie on your back with your knees bent and feet about twenty-four inches apart.
2. Rest your arms on the floor at a comfortable angle to the side and above shoulder height, palms facing up.
3. Inhale to prepare, and as you exhale, tilt your right knee down and in toward your left foot. The left knee remains pointed upward.
4. Firm your leg muscles, widen the back of the pelvis, then keeping the width, lengthen the tailbone along the same diagonal line as your thigh bone, toward the right knee.
5. Stretch your right arm along the floor and away from your thigh for a full connected stretch of the whole right side of your body.
6. Breathe fully, allow the ribs and waist area to spread, then release and repeat on the other side.

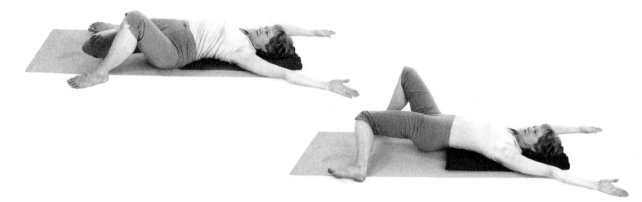

13. SETU BANDHASANA (Bridge Pose)

Purpose: To extend and strengthen the back of the body and open the chest and shoulders, extending the spinal range.

Contraindications: Absolute—Chiari malformations; Relative—sacroiliac joint derangement, scoliosis, facet syndrome, spinal stenosis, vertebral fracture, severe osteoporosis (risk of fracture).

Props: A yoga mat and a blanket.

Avoiding pitfalls: Keep the legs and feet parallel. Relax your neck, throat, and jaw as you breathe. If your neck is stiff, begin with a folded blanket under your shoulders and upper arms as shown. Avoid squeezing the buttocks too tightly.

INSTRUCTIONS:

1. Lie on your back with the tops of your shoulders on the top edge of the folded blanket and your head on the mat. Bend your knees, place your feet hip-width apart, parallel, and about six to eight inches from your hips.
2. Place your arms alongside your body, palms facing up. Take a few breaths, inflate your inner body, and soften any shoulder tension.
3. Inhale. Curl your sitting bones down and apart to ensure that the pelvis stays wide.
4. Exhale. Raise your hands until your elbows are bent ninety degrees. Point your fingers up.

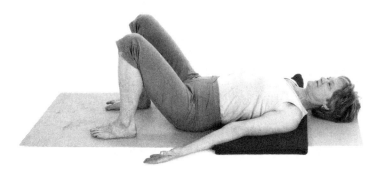

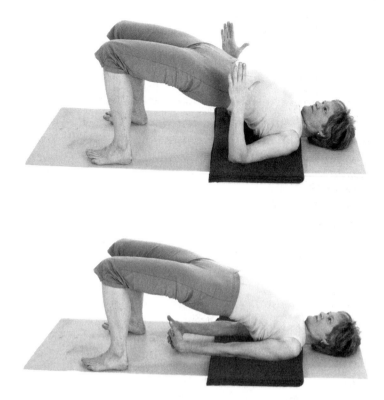

5. Lift your hips, spine, and chest as you inhale, then roll each shoulder under so that your weight is on the tops of your shoulders.

6. Point your knees straight forward. Lift and extend your tailbone toward your knees.

7. You can clasp your hands underneath you for more support, pressing the arms down to lift more. Interlace your fingers but separate the wrists.

8. Contract the buttocks, firmly lengthening them away from your waist without squeezing tightly.

9. Stretch the sides and the center of the body down from your throat out through the legs, unfolding your own power.

10. Exhale softly as you come down.

14. SUPTA PADANGUSTHASANA
(Leg Stretch with Belt)

Purpose: To stretch hamstrings, paraspinal and quadratus lumborum muscles, reduce spondylolisthesis and lordosis, and improve pelvic alignment. This pose increases poise and equanimity, while coordinating and loosening core joints.

Contraindications: Gastroesophageal reflux, hamstring sprain.

Props: A yoga mat, a belt, and a blanket.

Avoiding pitfalls: Keep the muscles of both legs firm and active, and the pelvis steady as the leg changes position. Relax your neck, face, and shoulders. Breathe smoothly.

INSTRUCTIONS:

1. Lie on your back with your knees bent, feet flat. Arrange the blanket so that the lower edge comes to the small of your back, with your buttocks on the floor.

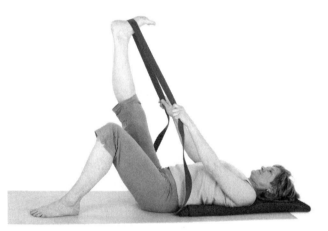

2. Relax and experience your body being fully supported by the floor.

3. As you inhale, move your sitting bones down toward the floor and apart, which will arch your lower back.

4. Contract your abdomen in and up and lengthen your tailbone toward your heels without flattening your lower back.

5. With your pelvis thus stabilized, raise your right leg and hook a belt around the foot. Hold one end of the belt with each hand.

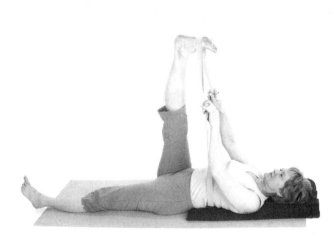

6. Gradually straighten the leg, firming the muscles on all sides and elevating your heel.

7. Adjust the angle of the leg so that you can straighten your knee. Use your thigh muscles strongly to fully extend it.

8. If your right leg stretches up to ninety degrees, then straighten the left leg to be flat on the floor for more challenge.

9. Extend through both legs fully, even if it means backing off with your right leg.

10. The main action is to push your right thigh away from your upper body (which keeps your lower back slightly arched) against the resistance of the belt (which pulls the foot the other way). Note: the goal is *not* to force the right leg or foot toward your head.

11. Once you have the actions, scan your body for unnecessary tension and release it.

12. Return to lying flat with both legs stretched out on the floor. Take note of any changes in sensation.

---

15. JATHARA PARIVARTANASANA (Reclining Twist)

Purpose: To mobilize the joints of the spine, strengthen transverse and oblique abdominal muscles, stretch the front of the shoulder, and strengthen the back.

Contraindications: Total hip replacement, colostomy, herniated nucleus pulposus.

Props: A yoga mat, blanket optional for comfort.

Avoiding pitfalls: Keep your muscles firm; do not do a floppy version of this pose. Align your spine down the center of your mat.

INSTRUCTIONS:

1. Lie on your back with your arms spread wide at shoulder height, palms up, and knees bent.

2. With knees bent, raise your thighs toward vertical, with the shins horizontal.

3. Firm your arm muscles, retract the upper arms back into the shoulders, and press the arms down onto the floor. The shoulders are the stable part of this pose while your legs and hips move.

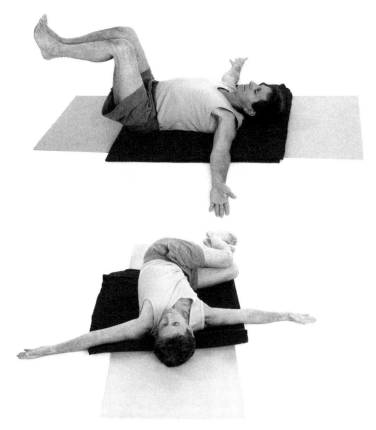

4. Prepare for the twist by first widening your sitting bones, then firming your lower abdomen.

5. Gradually lower both legs to the right, with the thighs at a ninety-degree angle to the torso if possible. Stretch through the lower back.

6. Press your right arm down into the floor and lower the left shoulder until it is flat on the floor.

7. Stretch your left thigh and left arm away from each other to intensify the twist.

8. As you get more comfortable (and more flexible), you will be able to straighten your knees in the initial position and throughout this pose. When preparing to twist with the legs straight, offset your hips to the left before twisting to the right.

There is a lot to keep track of in this pose, but the gains in range of motion, strength, coordination, and grace are worth it!

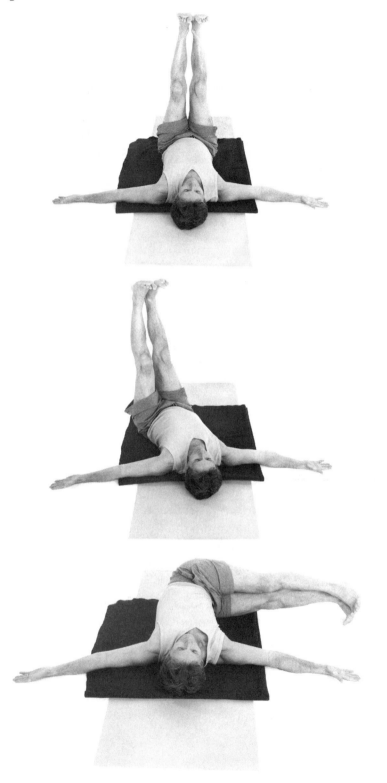

16. PLANK SERIES

Purpose: To strengthen the core abdominal muscles and the shoulders.

Contraindications: Colostomy, iliostomy, extreme hypertension.

Prop: A yoga mat.

Avoiding pitfalls: Avoid rounding your upper back toward the ceiling, raising the hips too much or not enough, or dropping the head too low. The body makes one straight line in the plank.

INSTRUCTIONS:

Stage I

1. Lie facedown on the floor.
2. Raise your head and chest up by supporting yourself on your forearms. Place the elbows under the shoulders with hands extending forward.
3. Firm the muscles of your arms.
4. Inhale and lower your upper chest down a little over the arms.
5. Exhale, contract your belly muscles, and lift your hips up to the same height as your shoulders. Knees remain on the floor.

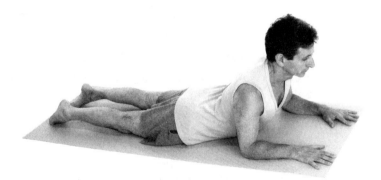

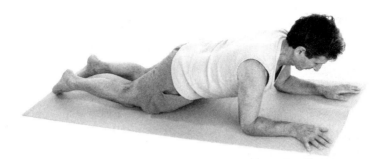

6. Hold yourself up just above the floor for several slow breaths, then release down.

Stage II

1. Perform instructions 1 through 4 as above.
2. Extend your legs back and tuck your toes under. Inhale to lengthen.

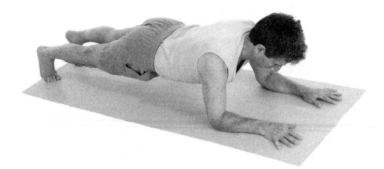

3. Exhale and lift your pelvis and legs up. Stretch and connect into one long line from shoulders to heels, suspended away from the floor.
4. Take several slow breaths, then release down.

Stage III

1. On your hands and knees, walk your hands forward about one hand's length.
2. Steady your arms, with elbows straight, while softening and lowering the upper chest.
3. Inhale as you lift your knees up and straighten out your whole body into one long plank from feet to head. Be careful to get the right

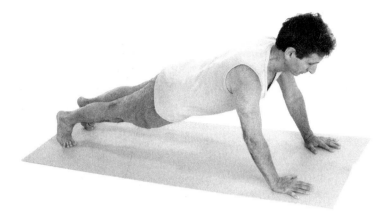

height for your pelvis and your head (the heaviest and least-supported parts, respectively)—not too low or too high. A friend or mirror can tell you.

4. Hold your belly firm and your legs active.
5. Reach the tailbone back toward your heels.
6. Be steady for several breaths, then release down with exhalation.

17. BHUJANGASANA (Cobra)

Purpose: To strengthen and extend the upper back and neck.

Contraindications: Fused ankylosing spondylitis, Chiari malformation, bridging spondylitis, cervical spinal stenosis.

Props: A yoga mat and a blanket.

Avoiding pitfalls: Keep your shoulders back and do not overuse your arms. If you get up into the pose and find your shoulders around your ears and your chest collapsed, come down and start over. This pose is about expanding the inside of you, and supporting yourself with the muscles of your spine.

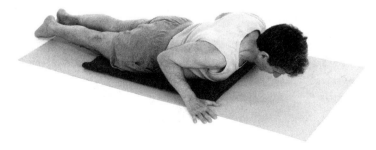

INSTRUCTIONS:

1. Lie on your stomach with a blanket placed under you for comfort.
2. Lift one leg up an inch and pull it back. Repeat with the other leg. This creates a good length in the lower back.
3. Briefly turn the front of your legs in toward the midline, so that the heels, thighs, and pelvis widen in the back.
4. Pull your tailbone toward your heels and toward the floor. This stabilizes your lower back, enabling you to stretch forward more strongly. The legs will rotate back to center so that the backs of the knees face straight up.
5. Lift up onto your forearms briefly to pull your upper body forward away from your legs.
6. Lie back down and put your hands to the sides of your chest, with your fingers pointing outward a bit and your forehead on the floor.
7. Lift your shoulders away from the floor, keeping them square across.
8. Inhale; lengthen forward through your whole torso. Expand from the inside.
9. Contract your upper back muscles and move the shoulder blades in toward the spine.
10. Curl up with your head and chest, keeping your shoulders back.
11. Press carefully down through your arms to lift more, but keep your arms bent and the upper arms and shoulders back.
12. Keep your pelvis on the floor while maintaining these actions. Use your breath to expand forward from the inside.
13. Stay up for several breaths, then soften and release down.

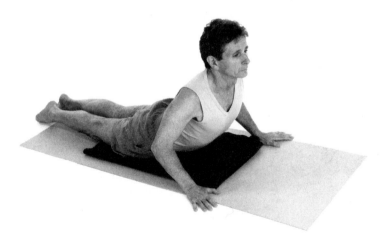

18. JANU SIRSASANA (Seated Forward Bend)

Purpose: To stretch hamstring, glutei, and quadratus lumborum muscles; to relax the back and improve hip flexion.

Contraindications: Colostomy, hamstring spasm or sprain.

Props: A yoga mat and optional blanket and belt.

Avoiding pitfalls: Keep the straight leg firm and press the back of the knee down. Move the upper body forward more than down. Bend forward from the hips as symmetrically as possible. Aim the navel toward the inner thigh of the straight leg.

INSTRUCTIONS:

1. Sit with your legs outstretched on the floor in front of you, with a folded blanket placed under your hips to make the forward tilt of the pelvis easier.
2. Bend your right knee out to the side and place your right foot against the inside edge of your left upper thigh.
3. Manually reach under your hips and widen the pelvis and upper thighs by pulling the skin and muscles back and out to the side. This will help you to tilt your pelvis forward.
4. Tighten the quadriceps of the straight leg, pressing the knee and thigh down to the floor, stretching the heel away from you. Evenly stretch your toes up and back toward you to complete the stretch of the back of that leg.

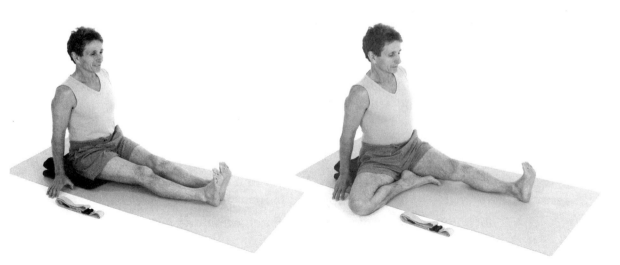

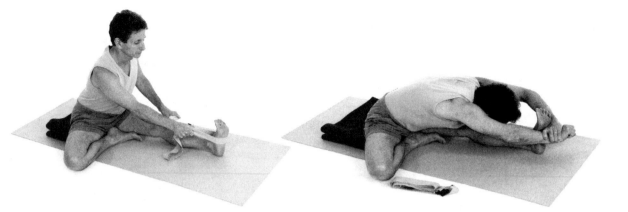

5. Press both sitting bones down and back. Inhale and extend up through the spine.
6. Exhale, with hands touching the floor, and turn toward your extended left leg.
7. Place a belt around your left foot and hold it with your right hand. The left hand on the floor will help you to lift that side of your torso.
8. Inhale again and stretch up again.
9. Exhale and bend forward toward your foot. Keep your arms pulled back into the shoulders even though they are also reaching forward. This will help you to extend the spine, refraining from rounding or collapsing it.
10. Shift your belly toward the left and try to even up the ribs, left and right, as you stretch forward toward your foot.
11. Use your breath to remain calm and avoid agitation.
12. If your flexibility allows, stretch forward fully over the extended leg, grasping the foot with both hands, or the wrist as shown.
13. Repeat on the other side.

Forward bends are quieting, once you get past the initial challenges of tightness. They encourage humility and patience with oneself.

19. CHILD'S POSE (Balasana)

Purpose: To passively flex the lumbar and extend the thoracic spine and flex the hips. To prepare for relaxation.

Contraindications: Colostomy, prepatellar bursitis, total knee prosthesis.

Props: A yoga mat and a blanket or two, possibly washcloths for the knees.

Avoiding pitfalls: If your knees are stiff, put folded washcloths behind your knees to create space and reduce compression there.

INSTRUCTIONS:

1. Come onto your hands and knees on a folded blanket.
2. If your feet or ankles are stiff, position yourself with your feet half on and half off the edge of the blanket. Place a folded washcloth behind each knee.
3. Widen your knees.
4. Fold your hips back toward your heels.

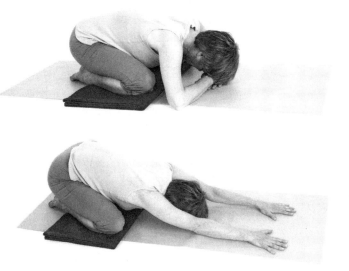

5. Reach forward with your chest and rest your forehead on your folded hands or on another blanket. An alternative stretch is to extend your arms forward on the floor.
6. Breathe deeply. Reduce effort and surrender tension in your body and mind.

---

20. SAVASANA (Corpse Pose)

Purpose: To relax, assimilate, cease effort, and consolidate gains from all the poses you have done. This pose is essential in making a safe and meaningful transition between the practice of the poses and the rest of your life.

Contraindication: Late pregnancy. Otherwise, dying is perfectly safe.

Props: A yoga mat, two or three blankets, possibly eye cover.

Avoiding pitfalls: After the initial setup, avoid fussing and fidgeting; become settled. Mr. Iyengar says this is the most difficult pose.

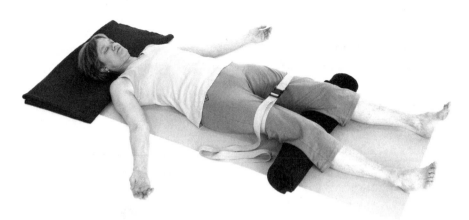

INSTRUCTIONS:

1. Make sure the space is quiet and safe from distractions.
2. You might like to have a folded blanket under your neck and head, a rolled blanket under your knees, and a third to warm you. An eye cover may help to relax your face and retreat from all outer stimuli. (See page 215 for use of belt.)
3. Lie on your back with arms at your sides, about twelve inches from your body with your palms up.
4. Adjust your hips by turning your legs inward to widen the back of the pelvis, then let the feet roll apart as you relax.
5. Lengthen the buttocks away from your waist if you feel any compression in the lower back.
6. Tuck your shoulder blades gently in toward the spine to open the front of the chest.
7. Make sure that your neck is long and your chin and forehead are level. Then guide your attention through your whole body systematically from head to toe and back again, letting each part relax deeply.
8. Do not fret if your mind produces thoughts; just watch them unemotionally without jumping into the content. Be a compassionate witness. You might notice yourself reviewing an event, thinking of a person, making a plan. Try not to follow the pull of the thoughts, but passively observe them come and go. Trust in the process of letting go.
9. After five to ten minutes of quiet rest, take a few deeper breaths, stretch your arms and legs gently, bend your knees, and softly roll to the side. Take your time getting up, to respect whatever effects, changes, and benefits you may feel from your yoga practice. Remember your highest intention and affirm your process of growth and healing.

All-Star *Asana*: Types of Motion

Name	Shoulder	Hip	Knee	Sacroiliac	Lumbar	Cervical	Thoracic	Hands	Feet
Tadasana	N	N	N	**N**	**N**	N	N		N
Tadasana Urdhva Hastasana	F	N	N	N	N	N	**N**	N	N
Tadasana Urdhva Baddha Hastasana	F	N	N	N	N	N	**N**	**E**	N
Standing Lunge with Wall	F	E,F	E,F	Nu	E				**E**
Adho Mukha Svanasana Series									
Puppy	**E**	**F**	**F**	**A**	**N**	N	E	N	F
Wall Dog	F	F	E	A	N	N	**E**	E	E
Table Dog	**F**	**F**	E	A	N	N	**E**	N	N
Adho Mukha Svanasana	**F**	**F**	E	**A**	N	N	**E**	E	**E**
Utthita Parsvakonasana	**Ab,R,**ER	**F,Ab,**ER	F,E	**Nu**	T	R	**T**	E	**I**
Utthita Trikonasana	**Ab,R,**ER	**F,Ab,**ER	E	**Nu**	T	R	**T**	N	**I**
Prasarita Padottanasana	F,**R**	**F,Ab,IR**,ER	E	**A**	F	E	**E**	E	I
Standing Lunge with Chair	D, R	**E,**F	**F,**E	A	E	N	E	E	E
Pressure Cooker	Ad	F,**Ab**	F	**A**	F	E	F	**F**	E
Chair Twist	E,R, Ad	F,**Ab,Ad**	F	**O**	T	T	**T**	F	E
Wall Quad	N	**F,E**	**F**	Nu	E	N	N	E	N
Lotus Prep with Wall	N	**F,Ab,ER**	**F,E**	N	N	N	N	N	E
Windshield Wiper	Ab	**Ab,Ad,IR**	F	Nu	T	N	T	N	E
Setu Bandhasana	E,R	**E**	F	A	**E**	F	E	N	N
Supta Padangusthasana	F,R	**F**	E	N	N	N	N	F	N
Jathara Parivartanasana	**Ab,R,D**	**Ab,Ad**	F,E	Nu	**T**	**N**	**T**	N	N
Plank Series	**F,R**	N	E	N	N	N	E	E	**N**
Bhujangasana	D,R,F	E	E	N	E	E	E	E	F
Janu Sirsasana	F	**F**, Ab,ER	E,F	A	**F**	N	E	F	N
Child's Pose	E	**F**	**F**	A	**F**	N	E	N	F
Savasana	R,D	E	E	N	N	N	N	N	N

A = anterior tilt; Ab = abduction; Ad = adduction; D = depression; E = extension; ER = external rotation; Ev = eversion; F = flexion; I = inversion; IR = internal rotation; N = neutral; Nu = nutation; O = open; P = posterior tilt; R = retraction; T = twist. **Bold** indicates intense action.

CHAPTER 6

The Shoulders

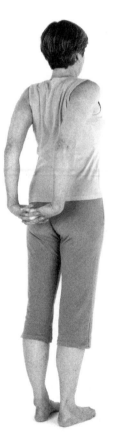

Most yoga postures or *asana* do more than one thing. However, the ravages of aging and the unpredictable events of life often leave an individual unable to do full postures because of disabilities unrelated to the primary goal of the position. Therefore, we have honed down some *asana* and focused as much as possible on specific joints to enable readers and practitioners to benefit exactly where they want to.

The shoulder is a particularly good example. Very little yoga is dedicated exclusively to this joint, though it plays a part in almost every *asana*. Some of the poses in this chapter are excerpts of full classical poses that offer specific benefit to the strength, coordination, and range of motion of the shoulders. The pure and simple nature of the movements, however, in no way substitutes for understanding the joint, which is crucial for getting the most out of our suggestions, as well as your shoulders. So let us start with a brief introduction to the anatomy of the shoulder.

The system of muscles, tendons, ligaments, and bones that make up the shoulder joint is unique. Although most bones connect to specific places—usually the ends of other bones—the scapulae, or shoulder blades, are different. They hang loosely and slide over a large region of the backs of the ribs. They are

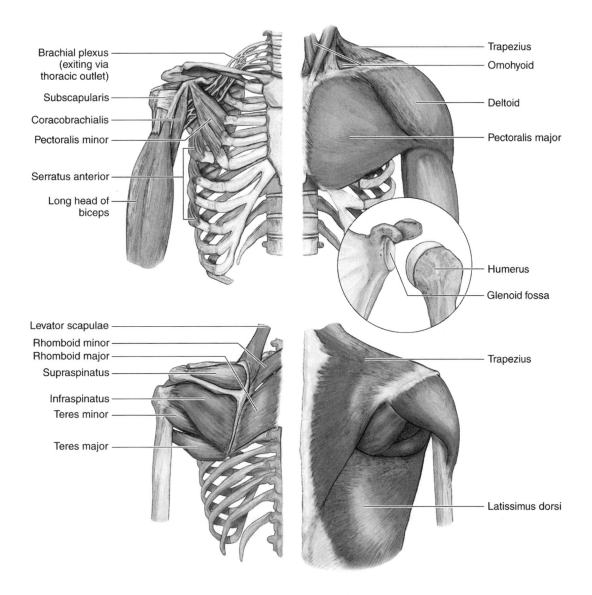

Brachial plexus
(exiting via
thoracic outlet)

Subscapularis

Coracobrachialis

Pectoralis minor

Serratus anterior

Long head of
biceps

Trapezius

Omohyoid

Deltoid

Pectoralis major

Humerus

Glenoid fossa

Levator scapulae

Rhomboid minor

Rhomboid major

Supraspinatus

Infraspinatus

Teres minor

Teres major

Trapezius

Latissimus dorsi

Figure 5. *The shoulder blade and the main muscles that control it and the arm.*

capable of rising, lowering, moving to the midline and considerably out toward the sides, and tilting in all three dimensions. The scapulae are not held in place by inelastic ligaments, as are the knees, hips, ankles, elbows, and vertebrae. Rather, a large group of muscles, each flexible and independently contractile, moves the shoulder blades or holds them in place each time the arms move. These muscles span an enormous spatial range in the body; they include the omohyoid and pectoralis muscles arising from the jaw and sternum, to the latissimus dorsi muscles that originate at the back of the pelvis. When you consider how moving the arms and shoulders changes your center of gravity, the activity at the shoulders is practically the whole body's business.

The shoulder's function is mostly related to supporting the arm and helping us do things with our hands, such as reaching and turning, twisting and carrying, and operating devices as various as a tennis racquet, a button, an automobile, and a scalpel. Sometimes the job of the shoulder is to hold things steady, as when you are taking a photograph, brushing your teeth, or performing tasks that utilize the fine muscles of the hand, such as typing. At other times, the shoulder does the lion's share of work, for example, when you are throwing a ball, where the hand only controls the release of the ball.

As osteoarthritis degrades the actual structure of the joint, encroaching at the edges of the glenoid fossa (the socket of the shoulder joint) or distorting the smooth spherical perfection of the head of the humerus (upper arm bone), the range of motion of the joint itself decreases. At first there is ample room for adaptation: the shoulder blade tilts farther forward or back, shifts up or down, angles right or left. This increased movement of the shoulder blade makes up for stiffness in the shoulder joint. The muscles that govern the scapula's position and orientation "give" enough so that the joint motions in question, those of the humerus in the shoulder socket, are not really challenged. But as the degenerative process continues, the ligaments and joint capsule begin to tighten, exactly because adaptation is so effective. A vicious cycle develops—the less the joint moves, the less it is able to move. There is no straining at the new limits on joint range; therefore, that range quickly decreases. And soon the easy adaptation stage is over, and the arm simply will not go up high enough to reach the top shelf in the garage, or will not twist far enough to hook on a brassiere.

The idea with yoga is to challenge these limitations before they outstrip your shoulder's built-in capacity to adapt to them. But this is not easy, precisely because of the joint's inherent adaptability! When you try to stretch the knee joint, you stretch whatever is stopping you, but when you do the same thing with the acromioclavicular joint, the shoulder will just slide along the back of the ribs to accommodate your limitation. So the exercises have to be more sophisticated, and have to fix the shoulder blade in place on the back of the chest before any of the shoulder's motions are extended. At times the poses cunningly do the opposite: hold the humerus in place and move the glenoid fossa around it!

The instructions in this chapter are drawn from Anusara Yoga as well as the teachings of Mr. Iyengar. What we have learned from Mr. Iyengar is implicit in what follows. Anusara Yoga explicitly offers four principles of particular value for the shoulder:

- *Inner Body Bright*—In preparing for any action, open to the breath, to your intention, and to a deep energetic expansion. Avoid beginning from a collapsed posture, both physically and mentally.
- *Muscular Energy*—The muscles of the arms activate, hugging the bones and connecting the upper arm bones securely into the shoulder sockets, which provides stability.
- *Shoulder Loop*—The shoulder blades pull in toward the spine and move slightly down, which causes a lift in the front of the chest. The tops of the ears tilt slightly back to maintain the normal curve of the cervical spine. This action brings the shoulder girdle and neck into an alignment that will provide both stability and freedom. Consult the diagram and explanation of the Loops in Appendix III.
- *Organic Energy*—While maintaining the previous actions, extend out from the center of the chest, out through the arms, creating space in the joints and balancing the compressive effects of Muscular Energy. With Organic Energy the practice becomes less mechanical and more expressive, fluid, and expansive.

Poses

1. WALL PUSH-UPS
(variation of Chaturanga Dandasana)

Purpose: To learn to maintain good support in the flexed shoulders while bending the elbows.

Contraindications: Severe wrist arthritis, severe rotator cuff syndrome.

Prop: A wall.

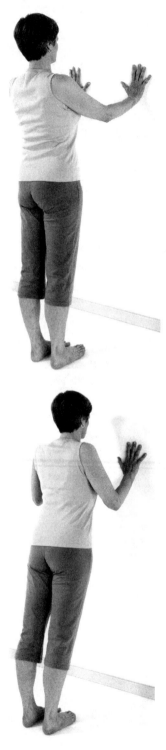

Avoiding pitfalls: Concentrate on maintaining the shoulder alignment, which should not be disturbed by moving the arms. Keep the shoulder blades pulled in toward the spine.

INSTRUCTIONS:

1. Stand facing a wall. Place your hands on the wall at about chest level, with your fingers pointing straight up, shoulder-width apart. Take a deep breath as you lift up through your torso with a feeling of expansion and readiness. Make the sides of your body long, from waist to armpits. Pull your shoulders back by contracting the muscles between your shoulder blades (Inner Body Bright and Muscular Energy).

2. Bend your elbows to approach the wall with your upper body. Move in and out, toward and away from the wall. Keep your whole body organized in one piece. Bend nowhere but at the elbows and the ankles.

3. You can coordinate your breath with the movement in a way that feels natural to you. This may help you to move more mindfully.

4. For more of a challenge, start with your feet farther from the wall.

---

2. SELF-HUG WITH BELT (relative of Garudasana)

Purpose: To stretch the outer shoulder muscles, increasing scapular range of motion.

Contraindications: Voluntary subluxation, posterior labral tear.

Prop: A belt.

Avoiding pitfalls: Keep your spine tall and your shoulders as soft as possible.

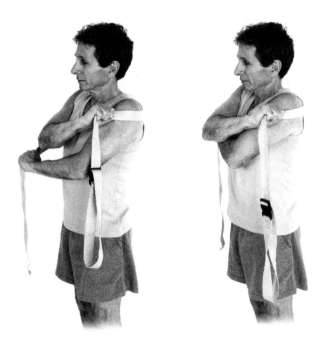

INSTRUCTIONS:

1. Wrap a belt around your upper back like a shawl, and hold it in front of you with crossed wrists.
2. Stand tall. Retract your shoulders, and firm your mid and upper back. Gradually walk your hands along the belt, crossing your arms in front of your chest. The arms reach out but simultaneously stay connected into the shoulder sockets (balancing Muscular and Organic Energies).
3. Lift your elbows up to shoulder height and keep a firm hold on the belt as you widen your chest from inside.
4. Repeat with the other arm on top.

---

3. PARACHUTE PULL

Purpose: To pull the trapezius muscles back and down, and to improve posture and reduce tension on the brachial plexus at the thoracic outlet. This pose creates a good Shoulder Loop.

Contraindications: Voluntary shoulder subluxation, severe wrist arthritis, suprascapular nerve entrapment.

Prop: A long belt.

Avoiding pitfalls: Follow the directions carefully. Do not cross the belt in front of your neck. The belt must be long enough.

INSTRUCTIONS:

1. Wrap the middle of a long belt around the bottom of your shoulder blades. Bring the two ends around to the front.
2. Loop the ends over the shoulders, cross them behind your head, and bring the ends down your back, toward the sides. Hold the ends.
3. Breathe, lift up from inside (Inner Body Bright), and pull the ends of the belt down. This will pull your shoulder muscles back and down, and help you to lift up the front of your chest (Shoulder Loop).
4. Hold for as long as is comfortable. Some like to attach the ends of the belt in front and keep the halter on while doing other activities.

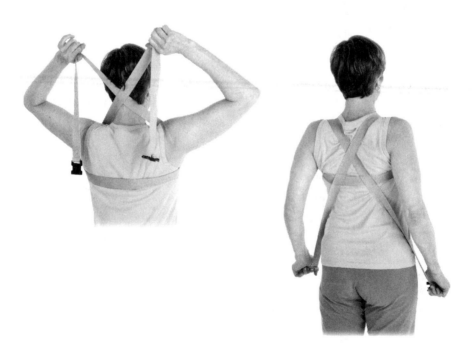

4. STOP (relative of Vasisthasana)

Purpose: To stretch the pectoral muscles, improving shoulder retraction.

Contraindications: Voluntary shoulder subluxation, severe wrist arthritis, Dupuytren's contracture(s).

Prop: A wall.

Avoiding pitfalls: Place your hand directly to your side on the wall, not behind you. Keep your muscles firm but not rigid, and your elbow slightly bent, not locked straight.

INSTRUCTIONS:

1. Stand with your left side to the wall, about eighteen inches away. Place your left hand on the wall, with the index finger pointing upward, the palm flat, with your hand directly to your side and not behind you.
2. Stand tall, especially through the side of the ribs. Take a breath to expand inside your chest with fullness and strength. Pull your left shoulder gently back and in toward the spine. Use a moderate amount of strength in your arm to press into the wall. Balance between the pull of Muscular Energy inward and the reaching out of Organic Energy.
3. Turn your body in place *away* from the wall. Stop turning when you feel a good stretch across your upper chest and shoulder.
4. Hold for a few breaths.
5. Repeat on the right side.

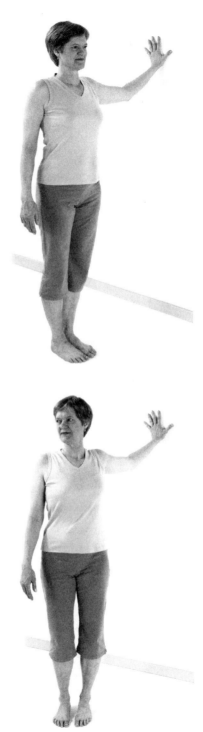

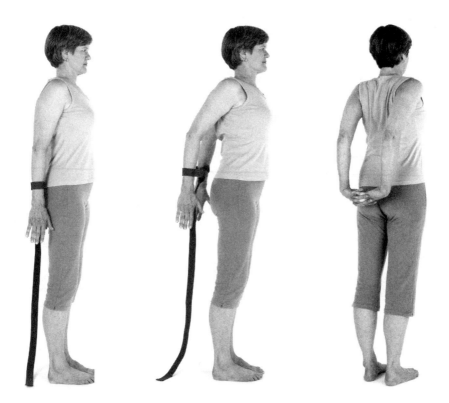

5. ARMS CLASPED BEHIND
(variation of Salabhasana)

Purpose: To strengthen the shoulder extensors and stretch the flexors, to improve posture and joint stability.

Contraindications: Recent rotator cuff tear, carpal tunnel syndrome (in that case, use a belt).

Prop: Possibly a belt.

Avoiding pitfalls: Lift your arms up an inch before pulling them back. Do not lock your elbows. If your back arches a lot, pull back through the sides of your waistline.

INSTRUCTIONS:

1. Stand tall, feet parallel and hip-width apart, with your hands clasped behind you or your wrists inside a looped belt.

2. Breathe in and lift the front of your chest, bringing your collar bones square across (horizontal) even if that means lifting your shoulders up a bit.

3. Strongly pull your upper arms back, rotate them outward, and push outward against the resistance of your hand clasp or the belt. Keeping your elbows slightly bent will help move the upper arms back correctly.

4. The shoulder blades will move back, together, and down. If your ribs go forward, pull back through your waistline to restrain the movement.

5. Hold the pose for a few breaths. Do so courageously, with vigor. Expand outward from your center.

---

6. CROSSOVER CACTUS
(preparation for Garudasana)

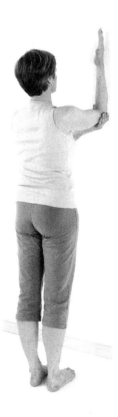

Purpose: To improve adduction by stretching the rhomboid, posterior deltoid, and subscapularis muscles.

Contraindications: Shoulder subluxation, acromioclavicular separation, posterior labral tear, Hill-Sachs deformity, or fracture.

Prop: A wall.

Avoiding pitfalls: Keep your arms back in their sockets and your collar bones wide.

INSTRUCTIONS:

1. Stand facing a wall. Lift one arm so your elbow comes right in front of the middle part of your chest, with the forearm and hand pointing upward.

2. Place that forearm vertically against the wall. Support the bent elbow with your other hand.

3. Inhale and firm your arm muscles, retracting your raised arm back into the shoulder socket.

4. Keep full contact with the wall as you turn

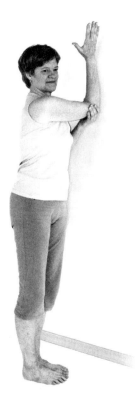

toward that arm until you feel a stretch across the back of your shoulder.

5. Adjust your feet to neutralize any body torque.
6. Stay in the stretch for several breaths.
7. Release and repeat on the other side.

This pose constricts the front of the shoulder, but stretches the back.

---

7. GOMUKHASANA ARMS ONLY

Purpose: To stretch the deltoid, triceps, and pectoralis, which are three major shoulder muscles, expanding range of motion.

Contraindications: Acromioclavicular subluxation, posterior labral tear.

Props: A belt, possibly a wall.

Avoiding pitfalls: Stand up tall to avoid distorting the spine.

INSTRUCTIONS:

1. Stand in neutral Tadasana, with your feet parallel.
2. Place a belt over one shoulder.
3. Raise your right arm in front of you. Turn the palm up.
4. Retract the arm back into the socket and raise it up near your ear.
5. Bend the elbow to reach your fingers down by the back of your neck. This hand will grasp either the belt or your other hand, which will come back and up. If you don't expect to be able to clasp your

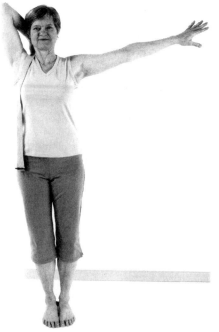

hands together, hold the belt with your right hand now. Then bring your left arm out to the side, turn your thumb down, and keep the hand stable as you pull the upper bone of the left arm back into its socket.

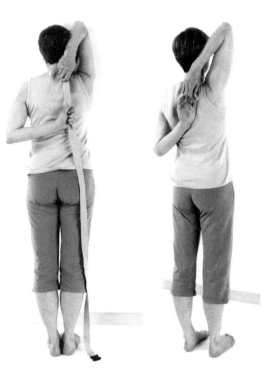

6. Bend your left arm in with the palm facing back. Reach up between your shoulder blades. Hook your fingers to catch the fingers of the right hand, or hold the belt.

7. Now that you have the basic shape, it is time to check yourself: Did you bend sideways? Do your ribs jut forward? Is your right arm as vertical as possible? The most difficult part is to get that bottom arm in toward the midline and up. Work patiently.

8. Hold the pose for a few breaths.

9. Gently release, then reverse the arms.

10. You can lean the right upper elbow against a wall for support, which takes some of the strain out of the pose and may actually intensify the stretch.

11. Again, in this somewhat constricting pose, work toward expanding from the inside.

8. PURVOTTANASANA WITH CHAIR

Purpose: To strengthen the arms and shoulders and stretch the front of the chest, improving shoulder extension.

Contraindications: Total hip replacement, inguinal or ventral hernia, lumbar spinal stenosis.

Prop: A chair.

Avoiding pitfalls: Keep your legs parallel, puff your chest out, and pull your shoulders back.

INSTRUCTIONS:

1. Sit on the front edge of a chair. Place your feet hip-width apart and parallel. Line them up under your knees, and then step forward one foot-length with both feet.
2. Lengthen up through the sides of your ribs. Pull your shoulders back.
3. Place your hands behind you on the chair seat, curling your fingers over the side edges.
4. Hold your shoulders back as you vigorously lift your hips up and forward off the chair. Stretch your knees forward as you puff your chest up. Look forward.
5. Make your body as long as possible from your shoulders to your knees.
6. Breathe strongly but quietly while in the pose, maintaining the lift from the inside.
7. Sit back down on the chair to rest. This type of arm-supported back-bending pose builds courage and stamina.

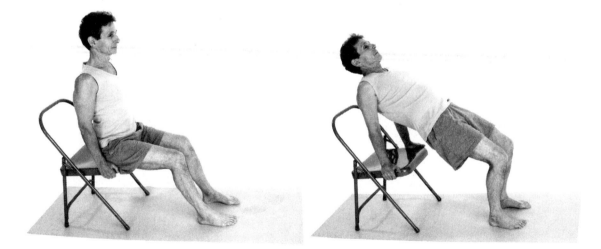

9. *ADHO MUKHA SVANASANA—See page 62.

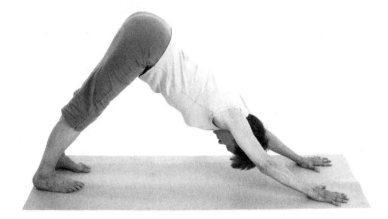

This pose stretches and strengthens the shoulders.

10. *PLANK SERIES—See page 87.

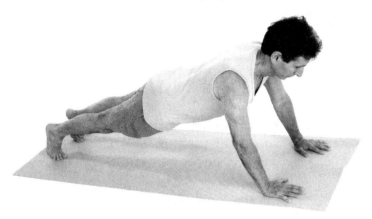

This pose strengthens the shoulders.

11. VASISTHASANA VARIATION

Purpose: To strengthen the stabilizers of the shoulder joint.

Contraindications: Rib fracture, severe scoliosis, severe osteoporosis.

Props: A yoga mat and a wall.

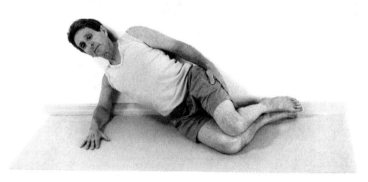

Avoiding pitfalls: Pull both shoulders back as you lift up. Trust your strength!

INSTRUCTIONS:

1. Sit on the floor with your legs to your left side and your knees bent. Place your right forearm on the floor, perpendicular to the wall.
2. Brace the back of the right shoulder. As you breathe in, turn your chest upward, stacking your left side over the right. Simultaneously

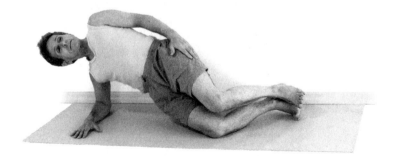

push down into the forearm and lift the shoulder and chest away from the floor.

3. If you feel strong enough and there is no pain in your shoulder, lift your hips off the floor for more challenge, leaving your lower legs on the floor.

4. Extend radiantly out from your core with full strength.

5. For still more challenge, lift the shins, fixing the body in a straight diagonal. Only the side of the one foot and the palm touch the floor.

6. Raise the left arm to vertical.

7. A wall behind you might help if balance is an issue.

8. Regardless of your level of elevation, do it on both sides.

9. For more of a challenge yet, see Vasisthasana Pose, Stage IV, on page 265 in Chapter 14 (Scoliosis). That version leads into the full pose from Downward Dog.

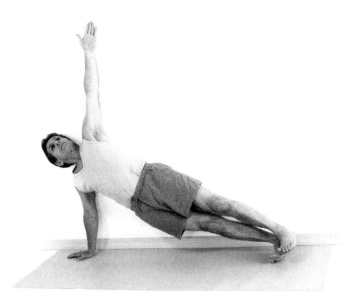

12. *JATHARA PARIVARTANASANA—See page 84.

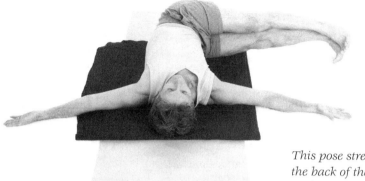

This pose strengthens the back of the shoulders and stretches the front of the shoulders.

13. *SETU BANDHASANA—See page 81.

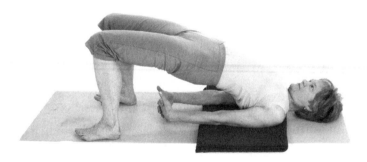

This pose promotes freedom of movement between the arms and chest, stretching the front, strengthening the back, and coordinating the two.

Shoulder *Asana*: Types of Motion

Name	Internal Rotation	External Rotation	Abduction	Adduction	Flexion	Extension	Protraction	Retraction	Elevation	Depression	Strengthen
Wall Push-ups					X		X	X		X	Serr, Rhomb, Tric, ADelt
Self-Hug with Belt	X			X	X		X	X			ADelt, Pecs, C
Parachute Pull		X				X		X		X	Rhomb, Lats, TMin, Tric, ITrap
Stop		X	X					X			Serr, Rhomb, MDelt, STrap
Arms Clasped Behind	X	X				X	X	X		X	Rhomb, PDelt, ITrap, Lat, TMaj, Ispin
Crossover Cactus	X			X[a]	X		X	X			Pecs, ADelt, C
Gomukhasana Arms Only	X	X			X	X		X	X	X	Delt, Subscap
Purvottanasana with Chair	X	X			X[a]		X	X			Lats, Tric, TMaj, PDelt
*Adho Mukha Svanasana		X			X[a]			X	X	X	Rhomb, Trap, RC, Tric
*Plank Series					X		X	X			Rhomb, Pecs, ADelt, Serr
Vasisthasana Variation		X	X[a]				X[a]	X			Serr, Rhomb, Delt, Ter, Lats, Trap
*Jathara Parivartanasana		X	X[a]			X[a]	X[a]	X		X	Rhomb, PDelt, MTrap
*Setu Bandhasana	X					X[a]		X		X	Rhomb, PDelt, RC,

ADelt = anterior deltoid; C = coracobrachialis; Delt = deltoid; Ispin = infraspinatus; ITrap = inferior trapezius; Lats = latissimus dorsi; MDelt = middle deltoid; MTrap = middle trapezius; Pecs = pectoralis; PDelt = posterior deltoid; RC = rotator cuff; Rhomb = rhomboids; Serr = serratus anterior; STrap = superior trapezius; Sspin = supraspinatus; Subscap = subscapularis; Ter = teres major and minor; TMaj = teres major; TMin = teres minor; Trap = trapezius; Tric = triceps.

[a]The glenoid moves over the humerus rather than vice versa.

CHAPTER 7

The Hips

In 1997, there were 117,000 hip replacements associated with hospitalizations for arthritis.[1]

Aging runners, soccer players, dancers, athletes of all kinds, and many who do not have a particularly active past find themselves unable to tie their own shoes, or find that walking, possibly just standing, or even riding in the comfortable seat of a luxury car for any length of time is painful. If they had an injury in the upper extremities they would have more leeway: they could turn the key with the other hand, move closer or farther from the easel, carry a package differently. But

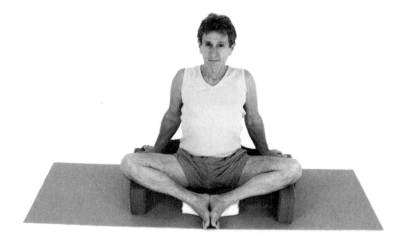

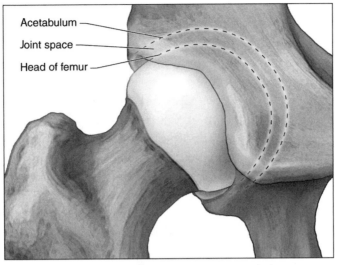

Acetabulum
Joint space
Head of femur

Healthy Hip

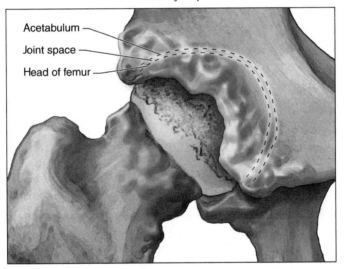

Acetabulum
Joint space
Head of femur

Moderately Osteoarthritic Hip

Figure 6. *Healthy and arthritic hip joints.*

walking requires the uniform use of all parts of the legs, and every joint in one leg bears all the weight with each step.

The architecture of the legs and pelvis is like that of a Roman arch, (see page 196), with the sacrum serving as the keystone between the wings of the pelvis and the femurs (the thigh bones). In a sense, the offset neck of each femur also resembles the flying buttress of a Gothic cathedral, a structure that parallels the joint's function: the femur inserts into the acetabulum, a socket in a thickened boney mass, maximizing the supporting role that the hips serve in us bipeds.

The femur moves in three ways: forward and back, away from and toward the body, and outwardly and inwardly. The symptoms of osteoarthritis usually show up first during adduction, motions of the leg inward, toward, and across the other leg. The first one is usually pain along the crease of the groin. Taking X-rays is still the best way to accurately diagnose and estimate the severity of osteoarthritis of the hip.

During the initial stages of treatment, nonsteroidal anti-inflammatory medicines, which come in a large spectrum of potency and safety, are often helpful in easing the pain and improving range of motion of the hip. After moderate progress and increased control of the center of gravity and hip muscles, the dosage can frequently be sharply reduced or the medicine discontinued altogether.

One particular thing to watch for in all patients with osteoarthritis of the hip is the combination of flexion, adduction, and internal rotation—the kind of movement required when you are tying your shoe. This is known to leverage the femur of a severely arthritic hip joint right out of the acetabulum, causing dislocation. This movement is generally severely restricted after total hip replacement as well.

Luckily, with yoga treatment for osteoarthritis of the hip, there are none of the problems that we had with the shoulder: there is no way for the hip joint's housing in the pelvis to move and adjust to the loss of range of motion. Here the difficulty is the opposite: in treatment the joint *has* to be made to increase its range, for there is no margin, no give-and-take, no flexibility in its set spot in the body or in its function. Anusara Yoga describes two beneficial movement patterns for the hip. They are spelled out fully in Appendix III. The goal of these actions is to center the femoral head in the acetabulum.

- *Inner Spiral*—The thighs turn in toward the midline, move back, and spread apart. This action broadens the pelvic floor and seats the head òf the femur back in the acetabulum. It also takes pressure away from the inner edges of the hip joints, where arthritis usually begins, and it arches the lower back, an effect which is balanced by the Outer Spiral.

• *Outer Spiral*—The base of the sacrum moves down and forward, and the thighs rotate outward. This action takes the outer thighs back, completing the effect of seating the head of the femur back. The lower back lengthens and the pelvis is stabilized over the legs.

Poses

1. CORPSE ROLL

Purpose: To loosen the hip joints and become aware of the range of motion for inner and outer rotation.

Contraindication: Late pregnancy.

Props: A yoga mat, possibly a blanket for head support.

Avoiding pitfalls: Work hard enough at getting the legs to roll, but stop short of causing strain.

INSTRUCTIONS:

1. Lie on your back, with your head supported if needed and your arms relaxed.
2. Separate your legs six to twelve inches apart, then relax them.
3. Slowly and easily roll your legs in toward each other, then away from each other. You do not need to pick them up off the floor, just roll them.
4. Picture the easy frictionless motion inside the hip joint.

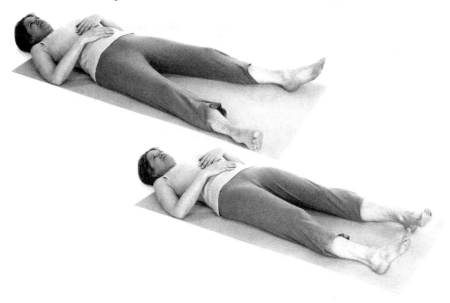

2. *WINDSHIELD WIPER—See page 80.

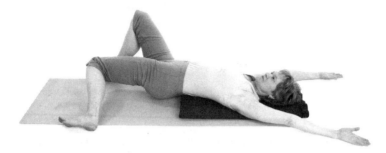

This pose is helpful in maintaining range of motion across the midline.

3. *SETU BANDHASANA—See page 81.

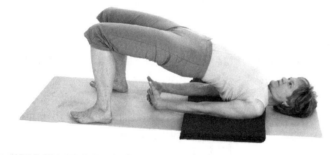

The legs are strengthened and the hip flexors are stretched.

4. *SUPTA PADANGUSTHASANA (Leg Stretch with Belt)

This is a variation of the All-Star pose of the same name.

Purpose: To sequentially flex the hip and stretch the hamstrings, improving hip range of motion.

Contraindications: Hamstring sprain, gastroesophageal reflux.

Props: A yoga mat, a belt, and a blanket.

Avoiding pitfalls: If the possibility of knee injury exists, hold hands behind thigh.

INSTRUCTIONS:

1. Lie on your back with both knees bent, feet flat.
2. Bring your right knee toward your chest with your hands. If grasping the knee is painful, interlace your fingers behind the knee to disengage the knee joint.
3. Carefully lower the left leg to the floor, extending through the left heel.
4. See if you can touch the floor with your left thigh; if you can't, gradually release the pull on the right knee until you can. Pay attention to the opposite actions of each leg: gently work to increase both as equally as you can.

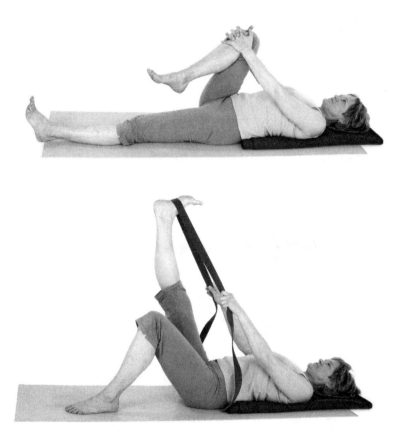

5. Maintain this stretch for a few breaths, then change legs and repeat.

6. Proceed to the instructions in All-Star pose 14, on page 83.

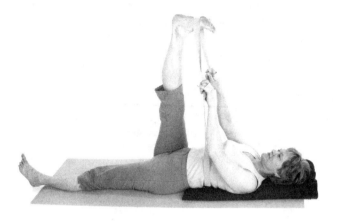

---

5. *LOTUS PREP WITH WALL—See page 78.

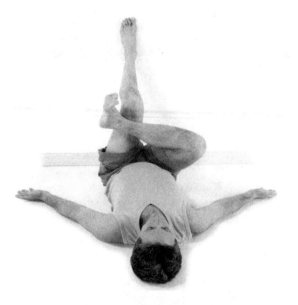

This stretch focuses on the back and sides of the hip joint. The support of the wall and the floor makes it a good preparation for seated poses.

6. BADDHA KONASANA (Cobbler's Pose)

Purpose: To stretch the adductor muscles, improve hip mobility, and coordinate these with foot eversion. To practice aligned leg actions that minimize foot strain.

Contraindications: Sacroiliac derangement, knee instability.

Props: A mat, a blanket, two blocks, and a towel.

Avoiding pitfalls: Begin using the props as described below. The props reduce the risk of mild injury to the lower back or knees. Progress at your own rate.

INSTRUCTIONS:

1. Do a test run to see what props you will need, as follows.
2. Sit on the floor with your knees apart and soles of the feet together. If your knees are higher than your pelvic rim, place a firm support under your hips until the knees and hips are level. When you are using a folded blanket, it helps to sit on the corner of the blanket, with your sitting bones fully supported but each thigh free from the edge of the blanket. This support will allow your pelvis to tilt slightly forward and your knees to drop lower. If your knees are high off the floor, support them with blocks as shown.
3. Place a folded towel under both ankles and heels as shown. This is important for the alignment of the ankle and foot. The ankles will be higher off the floor than the toes.

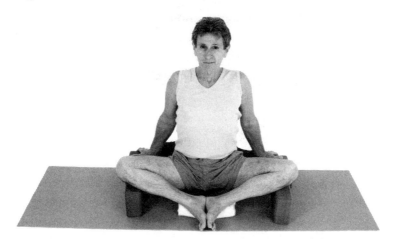

4. Manually widen your upper thighs and buttocks.

5. Place your hands on the floor beside you.

6. Take a full breath. Elongate and lift up your spine.

7. Firm your leg muscles, and do the following in sequence.

8. Widen the sitting bones and tip them back, which will tip the top of your pelvis forward (Inner Spiral). Walk your hands forward on the floor.

9. Curl your tailbone down and lift up through the abdominal area. Roll your knees more open if possible (Outer Spiral).

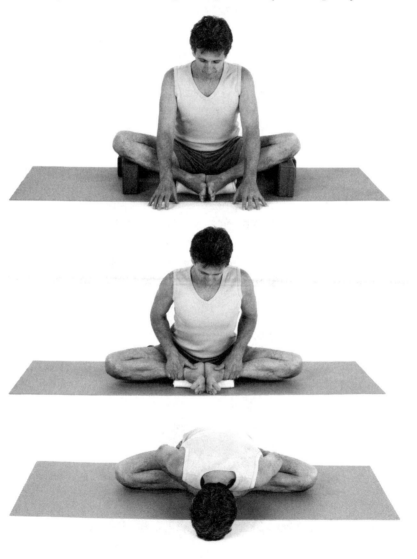

10. From the core of your pelvis, extend out through the thighs and up through the whole spine, still pressing your feet together.
11. To intensify: Hold your ankles. Lean forward, with your spine long and all the actions of the legs continuing. Isometrically push your feet into your hands as if to straighten your knees. This will deepen the hip stretch.

---

7. *JANU SIRSASANA—See page 91.

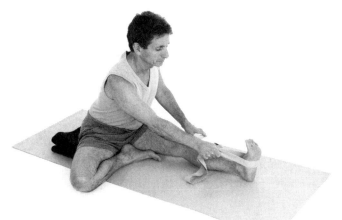

This forward bend stretches the back of the hips and legs.

---

8. *PRESSURE COOKER—See page 73.

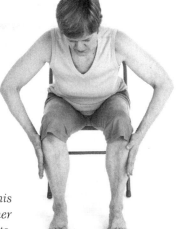

In helping to widen the pelvis, this pose takes pressure off of the inner edges of the hip sockets.

9. EKA PADA SUPTA VIRASANA
(one-legged reclining Hero Pose on edge of couch)

Purpose: To stretch the quadriceps and hip flexors one leg at a time, improving hip extension.

Contraindications: Meniscal tear, anterior cruciate tear, moderate or severe chondromalacia patellae, inguinal hernia.

Prop: A couch.

Avoiding pitfalls: Bringing the leg to the back in this pose will tend to cause the lower back to arch. To avoid that, flex your abdominal muscles and move your tailbone toward your feet. Also, stretch your spine up away from your pelvis.

INSTRUCTIONS:

1. Lie on the edge of a couch or low bed, with one leg off the edge.
2. Bend your knee and curl your foot back and down. Tilt your thigh downward as much as you can.

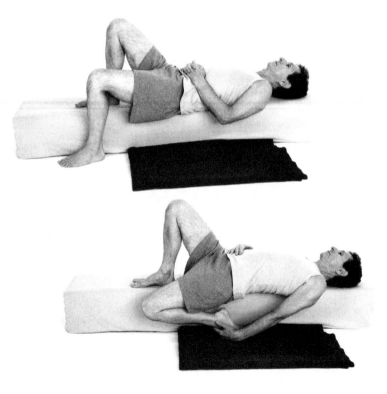

3. Reach backward with the thigh and foot. Align your foot straight back; tuck in the outer ankle.
4. Maintain firm abdominal muscles to prevent overarching of the lower back.
5. Use the center of your pelvis as the Focal Point: stretch out from there through your thigh and pelvis and up through your spine toward your head.
6. Breathe and maintain the stretch for as long as you can.
7. Repeat on the other side.

10. *STANDING LUNGE WITH CHAIR—See page 72.

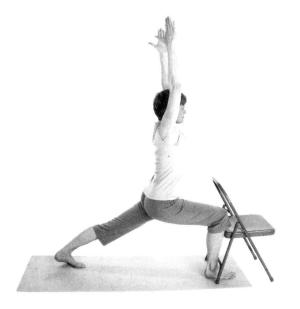

This pose opens the front of the hip, beginning with a chair for balance. Intensity can be varied by how the back leg is positioned.

11. SITTING LUNGE WITH CHAIR

Purpose: To safely stretch the rectus femoris, iliopsoas, and adductors, improving hip extension.

Contraindications: Ischial or prepatellar bursitis, medial or lateral meniscal or anterior or posterior cruciate tears, knee effusion.

Prop: A chair

Avoiding pitfalls: As in all hip extension movements, when the leg goes back, the lower back may arch too much. Work into it slowly, and contract and lift your abdominal muscles the whole time to support the lower back.

INSTRUCTIONS:

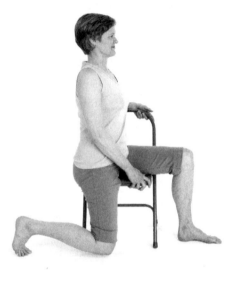

1. Sit sideways on the front edge of a chair, with your left thigh fully on the chair seat and your right leg hanging straight down off the front edge.
2. Lean forward and use your hands on the chair as needed for stability.
3. Firm all the leg muscles, and widen your buttocks and thighs, as in the Pressure Cooker (page 73).
4. Lengthen your tailbone down and lift your abdominal muscles up to stabilize your pelvis.
5. Once you are steady, carefully inch your right leg back behind you. The knee will remain bent as the thigh moves farther from vertical.
6. Breathe deeply as you reach back through the back leg; find the appropriate level of intensity of effort.
7. Stretch your leg back as far as possible. Attempt to straighten the knee.
8. Lift your torso up to vertical.
9. Enjoy this deep hip stretch, made safe by the support of the chair.
10. Bring the back leg forward to change sides.

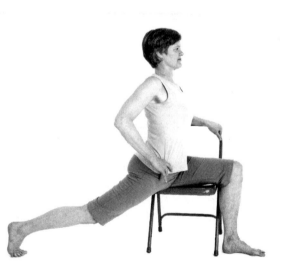

12. GOMUKHASANA LEGS ONLY
(with and without resistance from hands)

Purpose: To stretch the abductors and iliotibial band.

Contraindication: Ischial bursitis.

Props: A mat and one or two folded blankets.

Avoiding pitfalls: Use blankets under your hips to help you sit up straight with your pelvis vertical, not sloping back.

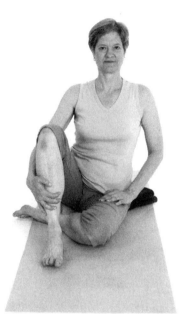

INSTRUCTIONS:

1. Place the folded blankets on the mat, with one corner pointing forward.
2. Sit on the front corner of the blankets as shown: left knee pointing forward, right knee up.
3. Grasp your right leg with both hands and cross it over the left.
4. Stack your right knee on top of your left, with the feet to the side.
5. If your knees stay very high up, use more support under your hips.

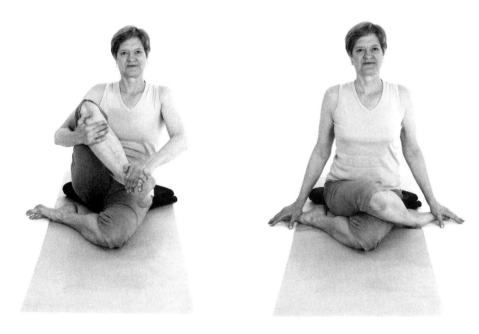

6. Manually move the buttocks apart as much as possible. This will free your pelvis to bend forward.

7. Inhale, lift through your spine, and tone the leg muscles.

8. Isometrically pull your thighs apart without changing their alignment. The resistance of your crossed legs will bring a stretch to the outer thighs.

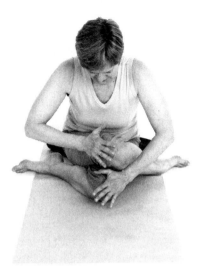

9. For more intensity, lean forward and put your right hand just above your right knee and your left hand just above your left knee.

10. Push in with your hands and out with your thighs for a stronger isometric action.

11. Breathe through your entire chest.

12. Release and unfold your legs to change sides.

The three standing poses that follow all stretch the hip muscles with the spine off center, promoting greater range of motion and strength and refining the actions of the hips.

13. *UTTHITA PARSVAKONASANA— See page 67.	**14. *UTTHITA TRIKONASANA—** See page 69.

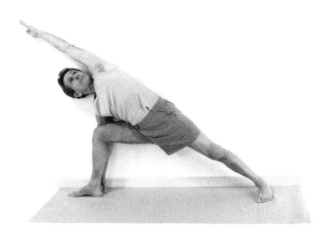

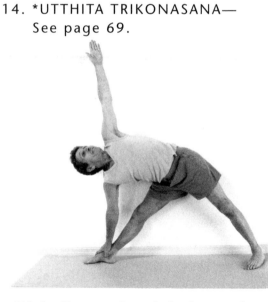

With the arm and leg extended away from each other, one side of the spine and pelvis gets a good stretch.

Side bending strengthens the lumbar muscles, while stretching the hips intensely.

15. *PRASARITA PADOTTANASANA—See page 71.

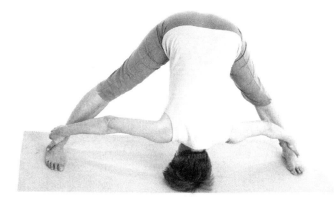

This hip and hamstring stretch is also a safe inversion.

Hip *Asana*: Movement Type and Intensity of Action

Name	Abduction	Adduction	Flexion	Extension	Internal Rotation	External Rotation
Corpse Roll					1	1
*Windshield Wiper		2		1	1	
*Setu Bandhasana				2		
*Supta Padangusthasana			3			
*Lotus Prep with Wall	1		1			2
Baddha Konasana	2		2			3
*Janu Sirsasana	1		3			2
*Pressure Cooker	3		1			
Eka Pada Supta Virasana				1	1	
*Standing Lunge with Chair			1	2		
Sitting Lunge with Chair			1	3		
Gomukhasana Legs Only		2	1			2
*Utthita Parsvakonasana	2		1	1	1	2
*Utthita Trikonasana	1	1	1			1
*Prasarita Padottanasana	1		2			

Note: Higher numbers indicate more intense action.

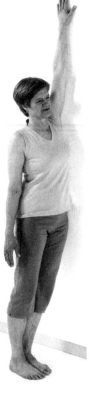

CHAPTER 8

The Lumbar Spine

Overview of the Spine

The articulated spine is made up of twenty-four distinct bones, or vertebrae, each linked to at least one other, or to the skull or pelvis at either end, with some adapted to link to the ribs in the middle. While they have a lot in common, different segments of the spine are quite specialized to perform their different jobs. The spine derives its virtues—its flexible support and resilience—from the summed qualities of all of its constituent vertebrae. But there are also great differences between them according to their form and function.

The five lumbar vertebrae, at the level of the waist and lower back, are large and thick, with transverse processes that permit the attachment of large, weight-bearing and weight-shifting muscles that support and manage the torso. Because these joints sustain considerable and abrupt forces, arthritis often begins early here.

The twelve thoracic vertebrae have flattened transverse processes at the sides, which connect to the ribs. The ribs and thoracic spine support the sternum, the clavicles, and most of the muscles involved in breathing, such as the diaphragm. Together, the muscles and ribs protect organs such as the heart, lungs, and liver.

The cervical spine's seven vertebrae are the smallest yet most specialized: the top two, atlas and axis in descending order, permit passage of the spinal cord and cradle the skull in a secure but highly

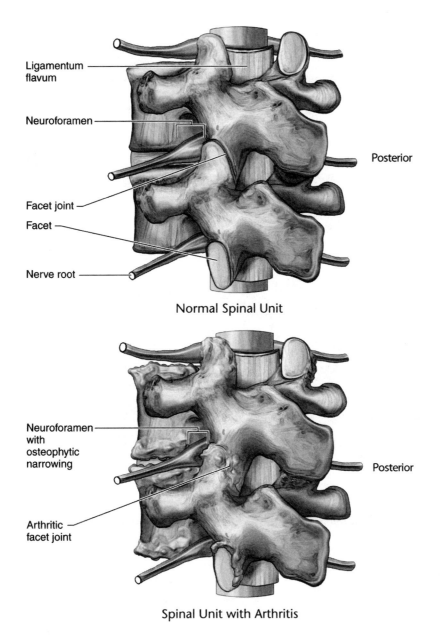

Ligamentum flavum

Neuroforamen

Facet joint

Facet

Nerve root

Posterior

Normal Spinal Unit

Neuroforamen with osteophytic narrowing

Arthritic facet joint

Posterior

Spinal Unit with Arthritis

Figure 7. *Healthy and arthritic lumbar spinal segments.*

flexible way. This arrangement, coupled with the five less specialized cervical vertebrae beneath the axis, permits quite an extraordinary range of motion to the head, enabling us great versatility in directing

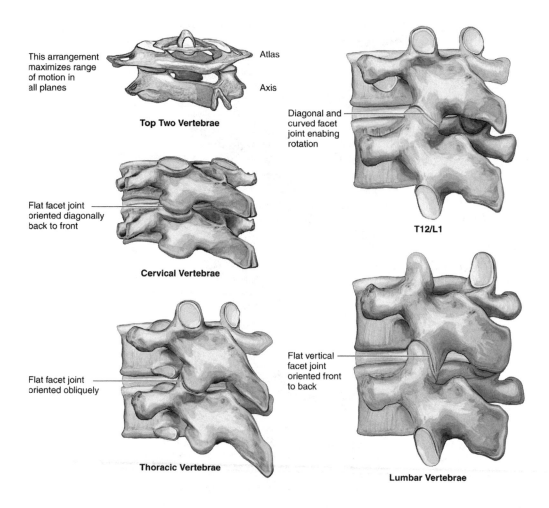

This arrangement maximizes range of motion in all planes

Atlas

Axis

Top Two Vertebrae

Diagonal and curved facet joint enabing rotation

T12/L1

Flat facet joint oriented diagonally back to front

Cervical Vertebrae

Flat vertical facet joint oriented front to back

Flat facet joint oriented obliquely

Thoracic Vertebrae

Lumbar Vertebrae

Figure 8. *Comparative anatomy of spinal segments: facet orientation in five different segments of the spine.*

our organs of sense and communications, especially our eyes, ears, tongue, and face.

The neck is a busy place. Nerves, the main passages to the respiratory and digestive systems, and great veins and arteries must fit in with, and coexist with, the many muscles that run from the head to the ribs, collarbone, shoulder blades, and the spine, the scaffolding that is necessary to mobilize the head. Arthritis affects all the vertebrae in some ways, but in the cervical spine, where space is at such a premium, and movement so essential, the swelling that comes with arthritis can have major effects on breathing, swallowing, and circulation to the brain.

There are spatial considerations all the way through the vertebral column, but once beyond the critical region of the neck, they generally involve the neuroforamina, the chinks in the spinal cord's boney armor through which nerve roots pass on their way to the limbs and other parts of the body. The combination of stress bearing and movement can result in the production of osteophytes, which narrow these openings, at times causing pain, numbness, and strange sensations called paresthesias, as well as weakness in the shoulders, arms, hands, hips, legs, feet, and sphincters. The facet joints bear a good deal of the stress, particularly when overweight or poor posture promotes arching, or lordosis, of the lower back. These joints are behind the vertebral bodies, bordering on the canals through which the nerve roots pass. Arching the back narrows the openings, and osteophytes narrow them further.

Other anatomical features that are not directly part of a spinal joint can also affect the nerve roots. The intervertebral discs often degenerate in the arthritic spine, which lowers the roof of the spaces the nerve roots pass through, the neuroforamina. Swelling of a ligament inside the spinal canal, the ligamentum flavum, can further constrain the passage of nerves just by taking up some of the unchangeable space within the bones.

With arthritis of just about every kind, extreme motion at any of the lumbar joints can compress a nerve root and cause pain. In addition, restricted range of motion even at one level of the spine puts more stress on the joints nearby, such as the hips, sacroiliac joints, and the shoulders. You might exhibit this extra stress by adopting unusual motions, such as when you are getting into a car or out of a boat or passing the sugar at a long table.

Yoga for the Back

Yoga may gradually improve the range of motion of the vertebral joints in all three planes of movement, increasing the ease and degree to which you can bend forward and back and side to side, and twist to the right and left. In doing this it is best to allot a share of the work of bending, weight bearing, and balance to each joint. If each of the twenty-five vertebral joints extends its range 3.6 degrees, that adds up to an additional 90 degrees of motion!

Yoga poses can also be directed specifically to the joints that connect the spine to the head, ribs, and pelvis. Greater range of motion in these joints has the same benefits, by "decompressing" the joints nearby. One prominent theory of osteoarthritis declares it the wear-and-tear disease. If that is true, then sharing the pressures and strains of movement evenly among more vertebrae has obvious advantages.

The same principle applies to the limbs. With more flexibility in the long muscles that cross the major joints of the arms and legs, especially the hamstrings, the wear and tear on the spine is greatly reduced. To appreciate this effect, think of the back strain people with tight hamstrings have when they try to bend forward. Expanding range of movement through increasing flexibility means greater safety for the spine.

First we will concentrate on the lumbar spine, then the cervical spine. We also include special chapters on the spondyloarthropathies that affect the thoracic spine, on the sacroiliac joints, and on scoliosis, which can appear anywhere in the spine.

Lumbar Spine

One key factor in preventing strain in the lumbar spine is to maintain its natural degree of curvature. Too much (excessive lordosis) or too little ("flat" lower back) is a precondition for arthritis and poor movement patterns. In both Mr. Iyengar's and Anusara Yoga, normal lordosis is maintained by balancing two actions: moving the top of the thighs back, which arches the lumbar spine, and pulling the tailbone down, which flattens the lumbar spine. We recommend that you determine the characteristic curvature of your spine in the spectrum from one extreme to the other. Do you tend to have a significant concave shape at the back of your waist, or do you tend to tuck your tailbone down and flatten your lower back? The best curvature is a happy medium between the two.

Anusara Yoga sums this up in three principles: Inner Spiral, Pelvic Loop, and Kidney Loop (see Appendix III). The Inner Spiral brings the thighs back and widens the pelvis, creating more lumbar arch. If you tend toward a "flat" lumbar spine, this is what you need. Conversely, if you tend toward an excessively arched lumbar spine, the Pelvic Loop (which lengthens the tailbone) and the Kidney Loop (which lifts the thoracic spine away from the lumbar spine) will help to create length and space there.

Other general tips related to yoga for the lumbar spine are as follows:

- In forward bends, be sure to bend from your hips, not your waist, and bring the top of your sacrum forward. Of course, tightness in the hamstring muscles makes this challenging.
- In twists, stabilize the pelvis in good alignment before twisting.
- In back bends, stabilize the tailbone and lift the middle and upper back away from the pelvis, to prevent all the movement from occurring only in the lumbar spine. This will coordinate the parts of the spine and distribute the stress of the movement.
- In any given yoga practice, do all types of movements: bend forward, bend backward, bend to each side, and twist.
- Be attentive to the neighboring areas of the body, especially the thighs, abdomen, and middle back, since immobility, weakness, or misalignment there can cause lumbar strain. The well-known advice to strengthen the abdominal muscles for lower back support is an example of this.

The poses here are arranged in three groups: beginning, intermediate, and challenging. How do you know whether you should start with the beginning poses, the intermediate poses, or the challenging poses? If you don't know what level you are at, start with the beginning poses. The intermediate poses are for people who meet the following three criteria:

- Their pain is below 5 on a scale of 1 to 10—that is, pain that does not intrude on your concentration.
- They have the ability to stretch the leg in Supta Padangusthasana (see page 83) to a straight ninety degrees or more.
- They do not have a history of back surgery.

The challenging poses are only for people who meet the following two criteria:

- Their pain is below 3 on a scale of 1 to 10.
- They have done the intermediate poses for at least two months.

If you cannot do all the poses in any section, bear in mind that it is best to do at least a forward bend and back bend, side flexion, and twists at each practice session. This thorough approach will also improve what we call "pelvic coordination," a combination of iliopsoas control, ability to widen the thighs, and an ergonomic distribution of forces in flexion and extension. While most people will be able to engage in all of the poses at the appropriate level of difficulty, the table immediately following the poses will help students and therapists choose the proper *asana* in special circumstances.

We recommend that people do beginning poses as warm-up for intermediate ones. We have made a list of poses from both of these sections as warm-up for the challenging poses. Our suggestions for this warm-up can be found at the beginning of the challenging section.

Beginning Lumbar Poses

1. *WINDSHIELD WIPER—See page 80.

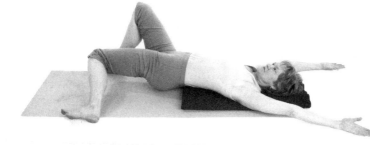

This pose is a gentle way to begin stretching the sides.

2. CAT-COW

Purpose: To mobilize the spine and raise awareness of the segments.

Contraindications: Spinal stenosis, scoliosis, spondylolisthesis.

Prop: A blanket placed under your knees if desired.

Avoiding pitfalls: Move at a moderate speed.

INSTRUCTIONS:

1. Come down on your hands and knees, placing them shoulder- and hip-width apart, respectively.

2. Breathe deeply to open up from inside.
3. With care but lightly, begin to curve and arch your back.
4. Inhale as you move your head and tailbone up. Let the middle of your back soften and descend toward the floor.
5. Exhale. Use your abdominal muscles to push your back up toward the ceiling. Let your head and tailbone curl downward.
6. Continue moving in this way for as long as it feels good.
7. Move your ribs and/or pelvis in slow circular patterns to loosen and mobilize everything, but go easy on the neck. You are warming up all the torso muscles and coordinating them—think fluidity!

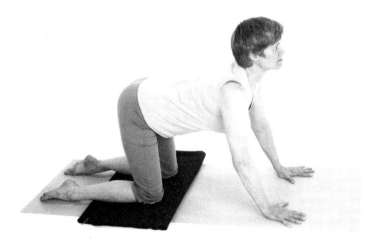

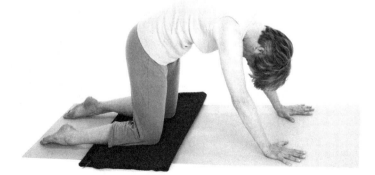

---

3. SIDE CHILD'S POSE

Purpose: To stretch the sides, enabling the whole spine to elongate, one-half at a time, facilitating lateral flexion.

Contraindications: Recent vertebral or rib fracture, scoliosis.

Props: A yoga mat and a blanket placed under your knees if desired.

Avoiding pitfalls: Extend and lift up both sides of the body even though the stretch will be on one side at a time.

INSTRUCTIONS:

1. On your hands and knees, using a blanket to pad your knees, sit back on your haunches.

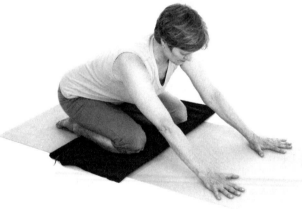

2. Creep to the right with your hands, curving your torso sideways. Maintain your legs in their original position.
3. Bend your right arm and place the forearm on the floor to provide a resting place for your head.
4. Stretch your left arm along the floor near your head. Curve it to

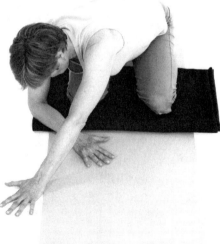

your right. Hold the hips and thighs steady.

5. Lift up the left side of your ribs and your left armpit to be level with the right side.

6. Find the longest stretch you can make; stay there as you breathe deeply. Extend out through your left arm and back through your left hip with a calm, steady effort.

7. To come out of the pose, raise your head and walk your hands back to center.

8. Repeat on the left side.

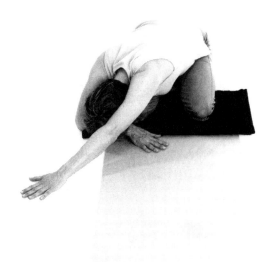

---

4. *CHILD'S POSE—See page 92.

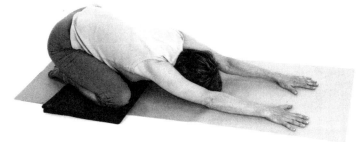

This gently curving stretch flexes the lumbar spine and extends the thoracic spine. It is often used between other poses.

---

5. *PLANK, STAGE III—See page 88.

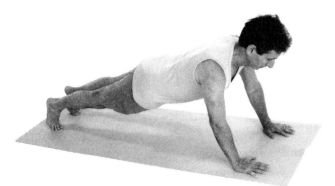

Strengthening the core abdominal muscles with this pose helps to support the lumbar spine.

6. *BHUJANGASANA—See page 89.

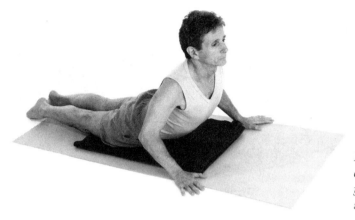

In this pose you create length as you arch the spine gently.

7. SALABHASANA (Locust Pose airplane variation)

Purpose: To strengthen the back's extensors, and improve posture.

Contraindications: Colostomy, spinal stenosis, spondylolisthesis.

Props: A yoga mat and a blanket under your abdomen.

Avoiding pitfalls: Come up into the pose slowly and carefully to avoid a sudden extreme load onto your neck or lower back.

INSTRUCTIONS:

1. Lie on your stomach on a mat, with a folded blanket placed under your abdomen to prevent lower back strain.
2. Stretch your arms out to the sides, palms down. Place your forehead on the floor.
3. Prepare the body with strength, drawing energetically into the core of your pelvis. Firm your legs and lengthen your tailbone. Firm your buttocks without squeezing them together.

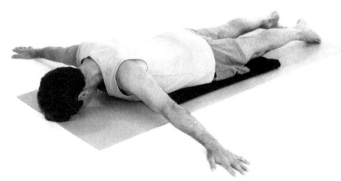

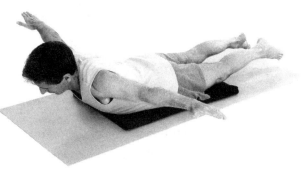

4. Lift the shoulders away from the floor without raising your head or your hands. Lengthen the sides of your body from your hips to your armpits.

5. Inhale and lift your arms, head, and legs a little off the floor, extending out from your center as you lift.

6. Stay up for several breaths, extending your upper body and legs in a continuous arc. Use the breath to remain light.

7. Slowly return down.

8.*ADHO MUKHA SVANASANA (Stage II, Wall Dog)—See page 63.

---

9. *STANDING LUNGE WITH WALL—See page 60.

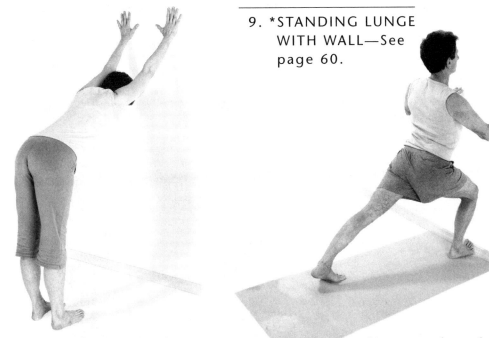

Here you lengthen the lumbar spine with support from the wall.

This pose stretches and strengthens the feet and thighs while safely increasing lumbar range of motion.

10. STANDING CRESCENT

Purpose: Mild lateral spinal flexion.

Contraindications: Vertebral fracture, rotator cuff or impingement syndromes.

Prop: A wall.

Avoiding pitfalls: Keep your body carefully aligned perpendicular to the wall. Avoid turning.

INSTRUCTIONS:

1. Stand with your left side a few inches from a wall. Lift your left arm high.
2. Test whether you are more comfortable with the palm side or the little finger side of your hand on the wall.
3. Firm all arm muscles and retain the upper arm well within the shoulder joint.
4. Inhale, lift up through your torso, and lean sideways toward the wall until your hip and possibly your shoulder area touch the wall.
5. Gradually intensify this side stretch during several breaths. You can step a little farther from the wall for a deeper stretch. Lengthen your sides.
6. Return to center.
7. Repeat on the other side.

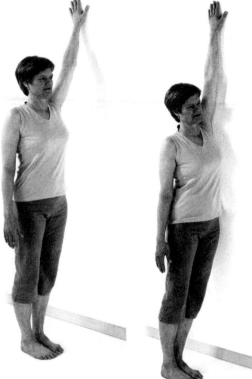

11. *PRESSURE COOKER —See page 73.

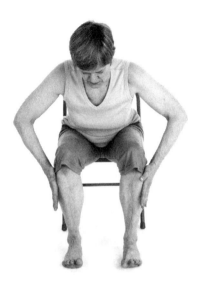

This pose widens the pelvis, giving more freedom to the lumbar spine.

12. *CHAIR TWIST—See page 75.

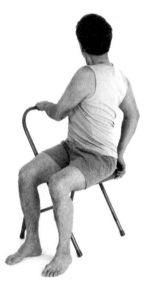

The chair keeps the pelvis steady so that the lumbar spine receives the benefits of the twist.

13. CHAIR MALASANA

Purpose: To stretch the lumbar spine's many joints in flexion.

Contraindications: Cerebrovascular disease, severe osteoporosis, vasovagal episodes.

Prop: A chair.

Avoiding pitfalls: Bend forward from the hips, not the waist. Reach your chest forward as you go down.

INSTRUCTIONS:

1. Sit on the front edge of a chair, with your feet parallel and a bit wider apart than your hips.
2. Manually pull your sitting bones and buttocks back and apart as in Pressure Cooker (see page 73).
3. Inhale, and lengthen up through your spine.

4. Exhale. Reach your chest forward and unroll your whole spine out between your legs.

5. Pull in your abdomen; breathe deeply; be sure to fill the backs of your lungs down to the bottom of your rib cage.

6. Allow your head to hang down. Touch the floor with your hands, gently retracting your upper arms into the shoulder joints while stretching your hands forward.

7. Breathe deeply and soften inside.

8. When you are ready to come out of the pose, reach your chest forward as you raise your torso.

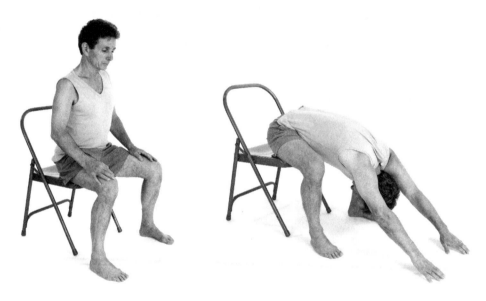

14. *SETU BANDHASANA—See page 81.

This back bend strengthens the back of the legs and the hips as well as the muscles along the spine, while extending the hips and torso.

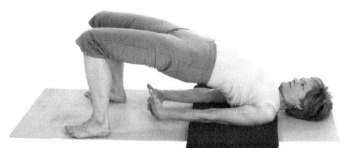

15. *SUPTA PADANGUSTHASANA—See page 83.

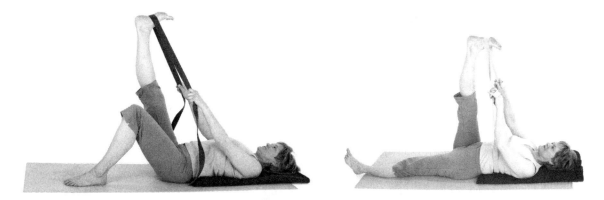

Here the hip capsule and hamstrings are strongly stretched, while the back is well-protected from strain.

Intermediate Lumbar Poses

1. *STANDING LUNGE WITH CHAIR—See page 72.

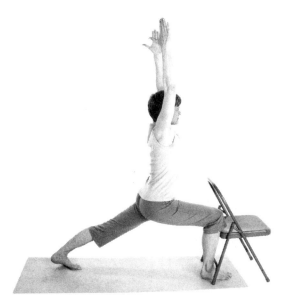

Like the Standing Lunge with Wall, this pose stretches the iliopsoas muscle, which is often involved with lumbar stiffness. The chair helps with balance.

2. *UTTHITA TRIKONASANA—See page 69.

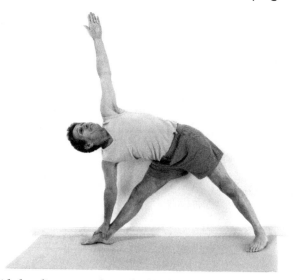

*Side bending strengthens the lumbar muscles,
while stretching the hip capsule.*

3. *UTTHITA PARSVAKONASANA—See page 67.

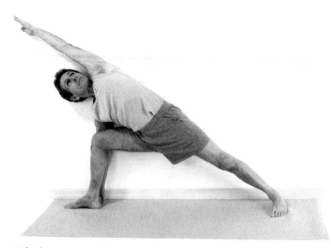

*With the arm and leg extended away from each other, one side
of the lumbar spine gets a good stretch. One hip is opened, the
other revolved, and coordination of the hips and lumbar spine
is improved.*

4. PARIVRTTA PARSVAKONASANA (Twisting Lunge)

Purpose: To revolve the entire spine and enhance range of motion.

Contraindications: Herniated nucleus pulposus, scoliosis, Hill-Sachs deformity, repeated shoulder subluxation.

Props: A yoga mat and a blanket under the knees.

Avoiding pitfalls: Keep the hips square to the front and use your breath.

INSTRUCTIONS:

1. Come onto your hands and knees, with a blanket placed under your knees.
2. Step your right foot forward between your hands.
3. Raise your upper body. Place your hands on your hips.
4. Inhale, firm your leg muscles to stabilize the legs, and lift up your torso.
5. Exhale, bend forward, twist, and place your left elbow outside the right knee.
6. Pull your right hip crease back with your right hand.
7. For the next few breaths, lengthen the spine with inhalation, twist more to the right as you exhale. Move into the pose more deeply with each exhalation.
8. Open your chest. Hold your head in line with the spine as much as possible. A combination of strength and softness is needed here.

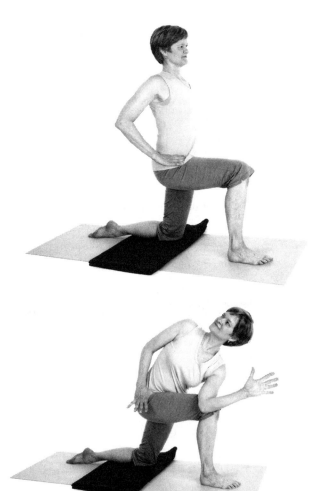

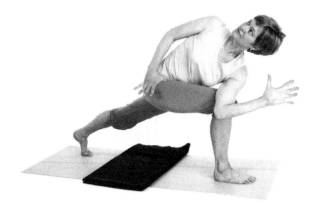

9. Return to center and repeat on the other side.
10. To intensify, tuck the back foot's toes under and raise the back knee. Straighten the back leg and draw every part of your body in toward the midline. Remain aligned from your head to your back heel. If balance is a problem, begin this pose with your back leg alongside a wall. Rise to the challenge!

5. UTTANASANA (Standing Forward Bend)

Purpose: To stretch the thoracic and the lumbar spine and the hamstrings.

Contraindications: Imbalance, retrolisthesis, hamstring tear, herniated nucleus pulposus, vasovagal episodes.

Props: A yoga mat, one or two blocks if your legs are stiff.

Avoiding pitfalls: Keep your legs working, whether they are bent or straight. Avoid letting the knees fall in toward the midline. Let your head release.

INSTRUCTIONS:

1. Stand with your feet hip-width apart.
2. Stretch your toes and lift them up, which activates the whole lower leg.
3. Retain the elevated toes and widen your sitting bones and thighs. You can lean forward a little to do this.
4. With the thighs still wide, pull your tailbone down and your spine up vertically.

5. Inhale and stretch up from the inside with full effort. You can relax your toes, but keep the leg muscles firm.
6. Exhale, bend forward, and touch the floor or the two blocks. Bend your knees if necessary.
7. Extend your whole spine from your tailbone to the top of your head.
8. Retain your arms deep in their sockets, even as you reach down.
9. For more intensity, hold your ankles and pull yourself farther down.
10. Balance your use of strength with an attitude of surrender and release. Breathe evenly.
11. To come up, first place your hands on your waist, then extend your head and chest forward and lift up strongly as you inhale.
12. Exhale and release your hands down.

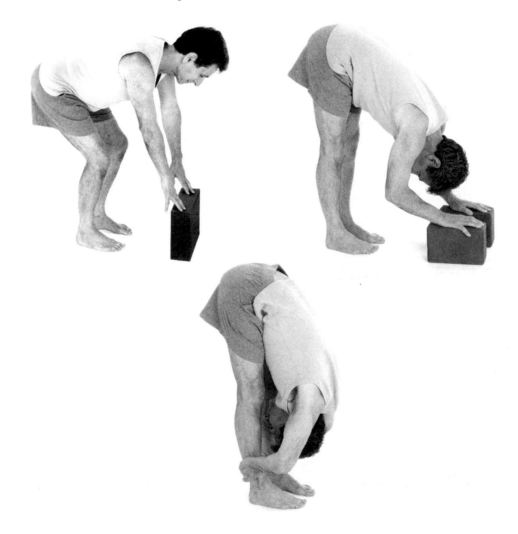

6. ARDHA BHEKASANA (Half Frog Pose)

Purpose: To stretch the anterior thigh, shoulder, and hip joints.

Contraindications: Knee effusion, tear of anterior cruciate or posterior horn of medial or lateral meniscus, rotator cuff syndrome.

Props: A yoga mat, a blanket for padding if desired.

Avoiding pitfalls: Keep the spine long and the bending leg close in to the midline. If you have lumbar or thoracolumbar scoliosis, then do this pose only on the convex side.

INSTRUCTIONS:

1. Lie on your stomach.
2. Prepare by lengthening: pull your ribs forward away from the pelvis and stretch your legs back.
3. Come up onto your right forearm.
4. Bend your left knee and grasp your left arch with your left hand, with the palm facing to the left.
5. Spread your toes, especially the fourth and fifth ones. This will help to protect your knee.
6. Press the left knee down toward the floor to soften the groin.
7. Then press the tailbone down and pull your foot down and toward the outside of your hip.
8. Symmetrically extend your torso up and forward. This involves more stretching on the left side. Pull the left shoulder up and back as much as you can.
9. With your awareness and effort spread evenly through your body, maintain the pose for several breaths, then release and repeat on the other side.

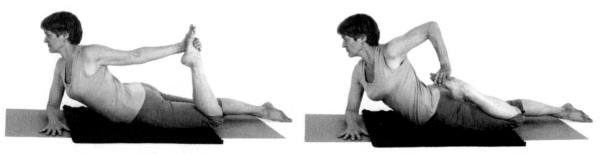

7. USTRASANA WITH CHAIR (Camel Pose)

Purpose: To strengthen the spine, increase its arch, strengthen the legs, and improve posture.

Contraindications: Spinal stenosis, spondylolisthesis, recent abdominal surgery.

Props: A blanket and a chair.

Avoiding pitfalls: Lift up strongly before arching your back.

INSTRUCTIONS:

1. Kneel with your back to a chair, with your legs hip-width apart and your feet under the chair seat.
2. Align your calves and feet straight back and parallel.
3. Lean forward slightly and widen your thighs apart, as in Pressure Cooker (see page 73).
4. Come upright again and pull your tailbone down.
5. Lift up through the mid-torso, but hold the sides of the waist back. This is Anusara Yoga's Kidney Loop (see Appendix III). It helps to prevent compression of the lumbar vertebrae during back bends.
6. Retract your shoulder blades toward the spine and begin to reach your arms behind you.
7. Inhale and vigorously lift your heart.
8. Reach for the chair seat or legs with your hands. Slowly and sequentially arch your midback, upper back, and chest.

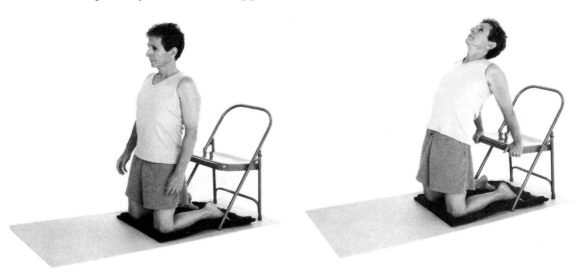

9. Move your ears back, then slowly arch your neck and head back.
10. These things will support and guide you; your lower legs press into the floor, your tailbone presses forward, your heart lifts up, and your breathing centers you.
11. To exit the pose, lift your head and shoulders upright, then sit down on your heels.

---

8. PARIGHASANA WITH CHAIR (Gate Lock Pose)

Purpose: To laterally stretch the torso and one leg, improving lateral flexion.

Contraindications: Herniated nucleus pulposus, facet syndrome.

Props: A yoga mat, a blanket placed under the knee and heel, and a chair.

Avoiding pitfalls: Stretch upward before bending to the side. If you have lumbar or thoracolumbar scoliosis, lean only to the convex side.

INSTRUCTIONS:

1. Spread a blanket on the mat and place a chair at one end.
2. Kneel with the chair off to the right. Point your feet straight back behind you.

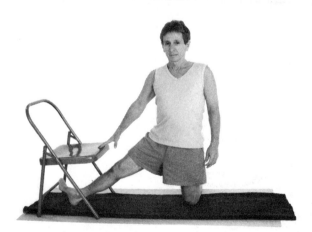

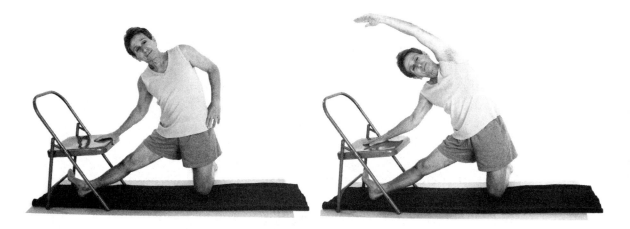

3. Extend your right leg diagonally to the side, with the heel down and toes up. Place your right foot under the chair seat. Your right hand rests on the chair seat, your left hand on your hip.

4. Keep your left hip and knee aligned vertically.

5. With a deep breath in, firm your leg muscles and lengthen through your spine. Pull your shoulders back.

6. Exhale and curve your spine to the right.

7. For more intensity, stretch your left arm overhead with the palm facing to the right and down.

8. Maintain a stretch through your legs, spine, and arms for a few breaths. Extend from the core of your body out to the periphery.

9. Inhale as you come up, then repeat on the other side.

9. PIGEON POSE WITH BOLSTER AND CHAIR

Purpose: To stretch the anterior hip and improve extension.

Contraindications: Prepatellar bursitis, spinal stenosis, recent abdominal surgery, hernias, facet syndrome (segmental rigidity).

Props: A bolster, blanket(s), and a chair.

Avoiding pitfalls: Face your hips squarely to the chair, with your forward leg open to the side and the back leg going straight behind you. Add a folded blanket on top of the bolster if your hips are stiff.

INSTRUCTIONS:

1. Place a bolster about twelve to sixteen inches from the front of the chair.
2. Position yourself onto the bolster, with your right leg in front and left leg behind.
3. Bend your right knee out to the side.
4. Stretch your left leg straight back, with the kneecap and toes facing down.
5. Support yourself with your forearms in the chair seat.
6. Check that your pelvis is facing straight forward. Pull your left hip forward if necessary to achieve it.
7. Firm your leg muscles.
8. Isometrically abduct your upper thighs away from the midline.

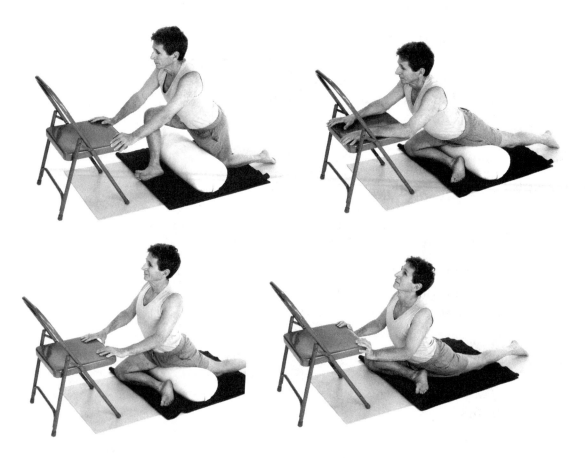

9. Curl your tailbone down and lift your abdomen up.
10. Without turning your pelvis, settle it down as much as possible; slide the back leg farther back if you can.
11. Stretch out through the back leg and up through your entire spine. Continue to face the chair directly.
12. For more intensity, take the bolster out and arch up through your upper back and neck. You can press on the chair for more lift.
13. Take several breaths. Lift your chest while rooting the hips down. Remain poised in the midline for this asymmetrical pose.
14. Release and repeat on the other side.

10. *JANU SIRSASANA — See page 91.

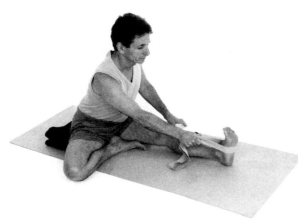

This is a good stretch of the lumbar muscles in a forward bend.

11. *CHILD'S POSE—See page 92.

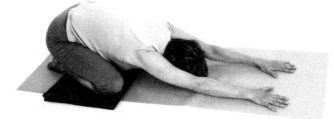

This pose is a gentle ending to the sequence.

Challenging Lumbar Poses

We recommend that you do a warm-up sequence of twelve poses from the beginning and intermediate sections, in the following order: Cat-Cow, Side Child, Bhujangasana, Ardha Bhekasana, Adho Mukha Svanasana, Pressure Cooker, Chair Twist, Parighasana, Ustrasana, Utthita Parsvakonasana, Utthita Trikonasana, and Uttanasana.

1. VIPARITA DANDASANA PREP
(Supported Back Bend with Chair and Wall)

Purpose: To stretch the abdominal muscles and hip flexors and extend the spine.

Contraindications: Recent abdominal surgery, spinal stenosis.

Props: A folding chair, a wall, and a blanket. Cushions if desired.

Avoiding pitfalls: Adjust your position in the chair relative to your height. Taller people will sit farther into the chair in the beginning. Take care to lengthen your back as you arch into the full pose.

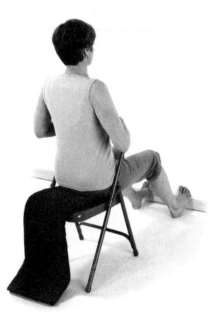

INSTRUCTIONS:

1. Place your chair about two feet from a wall. Place a folded blanket on the seat.
2. Sit backward in the chair, on the edge of a blanket, with your legs threaded through the backrest.
3. Bring your toes up the wall while your heels are on the floor and your knees are bent.
4. Manually widen your sitting bones and upper thighs.
5. Firm and lift your abdominal muscles.
6. Hold the sides of the chair back with your hands.
7. Inhaling, lift your back ribs up and bow forward, rounding your spine slightly. This is the Kidney Loop again (see Appendix III).

8. Exhale and start to lean back, still rounding your back to create length, until your upper back reaches the front edge of the chair. Come farther into the chair with your hips if you need to, in order to have the spine just below the shoulder blades come to the edge of the chair.

9. Once your back is on the chair and before moving your shoulders and neck into a deeper arch, firm your shoulder blades onto your back and lift your heart up.

10. Move the sides of your neck back and up, lengthening the neck before arching it.

11. Exhale, and arch back with your shoulders and head over the front of the chair. Rest your head on a pile of cushions, or let it hang if

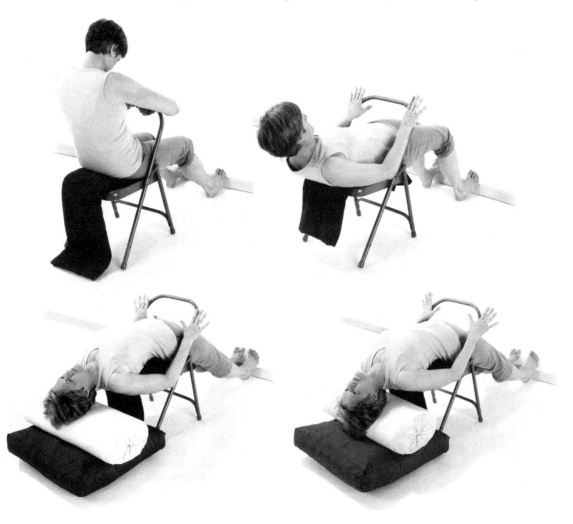

this is comfortable. Your hands can stay on the backrest, and even push lightly to increase the opening of your chest.

12. Push into the wall with your feet, straightening your legs. The chair may slide away from the wall a little. Use that action of your legs to support a large expansion in your chest as it arches back.

13. Extend through the whole length of your body. Let inside and outside merge as you breathe fully.

14. To come up, bend your knees and slide back to plant your hips firmly on the chair. Keep your chest open; use your arms to lift your chest.

15. Sit upright for a few breaths to rest before coming out of the chair.

6. SUPTA VIRASANA (Reclining Hero Pose)

Purpose: To stretch the thighs, knees, and hip flexors.

Contraindication: Knee pathology.

Props: A block, a bolster, several blankets, and two washcloths.

Avoiding pitfalls: Take care to use enough props to avoid straining the knees or lower back. Take note of instructions and pictures for prop use. If difficulties ensue, consult a teacher.

INSTRUCTIONS:

1. Set up the block and the bolster lengthwise on a mat, with a blanket placed beneath them for padding. Have another blanket or two ready.

2. Sit on the block with your feet folded to the outsides of your hips, and knees straight forward. If your knees are uncomfortable, add one folded blanket under your hips and washcloths at the back of the knees. If you need less support, remove the block or use a folded blanket under your hips.

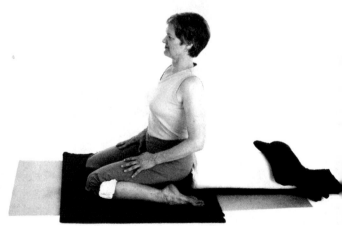

3. Adjust the leg muscles with your hands: buttocks wider, thighs turned in, and calf muscles away from the knees.
4. Set one other folded blanket or more behind you to support your back and head as you lie down. If you feel stiffness or pain in your knees or lower back, stack these blankets over the bolster for more height.
5. Inhale, lift your spine and ribs, and lower your tailbone.
6. Start leaning back, support yourself on your arms, and lengthen the lower back as you go.

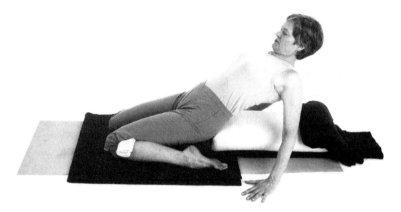

7. As you descend and arrive on the blankets, pull your lower ribs away from your waistline to maximize the length of your back, stretch your tailbone toward your knees, and keep your abdominal muscles pulling in and up.
8. An intense thigh stretch is good, but knee or lower back pain is not good. Adjust with more height under you if necessary.

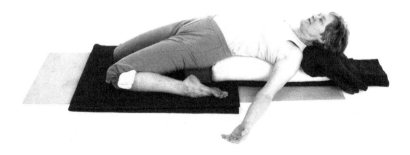

9. Stay in the pose for a minute or two, focusing on creating inner length and inner calm, and then come up and roll to one side to release your legs.

---

3. PARIVRTTA JANU SIRSASANA
(Revolved Head to Knee Pose)

Purpose: To stretch the legs, hips, and side of the torso.

Contraindications: Absolute: pregnancy. Relative: fractured vertebra or rib, colostomy. With scoliosis, do this pose only when the leg on the convex side is straight. Refrain from doing this pose on the other side.

Props: A mat and possibly a belt.

Avoiding pitfalls: Go into the pose in several careful stages.

INSTRUCTIONS:

1. Sit with your legs extended forward in front of you.
2. Pull your left knee out to the side and back, folding the foot in close to you. Separate the thighs as widely as possible.
3. Turn toward your left and extend your spine up.
4. Firm your legs, stretching out through your right heel.
5. Inhale, stretch your spine up, exhale, and incline toward your right leg.
6. Pause here and root your right thigh down to keep the knee straight.

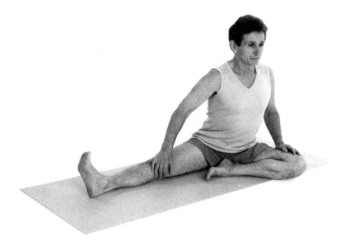

7. On another exhalation, curve your body over to the right, your right arm coming alongside your right leg.

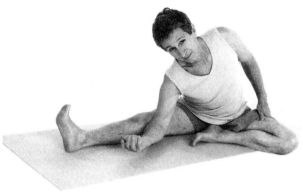

8. Reach for the right foot with your hand. Turn your palm up. Use a belt if necessary.

9. Turn your left ribs up and back as the right side comes forward to twist the spine.

10. Sweep your left hand out, up overhead, and to the right to grasp the right toes if possible. If not, reach up and over with the left arm to stretch your left side.

11. Let your breath and your intention for healing lead you into this deep side stretch.

12. When you are ready to come up, root down through the pelvis and legs and inhale strongly as you rise. Repeat on the second side.

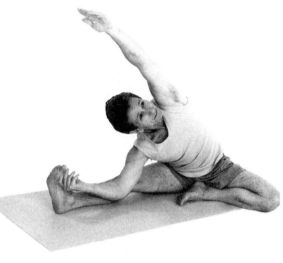

4. BHARADVAJASANA

This twist is dedicated to Bharadvaja, a hero from the Mahabharata.

Purpose: To improve a critical range of motion in the spine and stretch the outer parts of the hips as well, one at a time.

Contraindications: Absolute: pregnancy. Relative: herniated nucleus pulposus, total hip replacement, colostomy.

Props: A yoga mat and a folded blanket.

Avoiding pitfalls: Use enough support under your hips to orient your pelvis vertically (without tipping back) and place both knees on the floor.

INSTRUCTIONS:

1. Sit next to the blanket with your legs folded under you.
2. Move your hips to the right, settling your right hip onto the corner of a folded blanket.
3. Your feet are to the left, with the right instep in the arch of the left foot.
4. Manually pull your buttocks back and apart.
5. Inhale and stretch up through your spine. Retract your abdomen.
6. Exhale as you turn to your right. Reach your right hand behind you on the floor; place your left hand on your right knee.

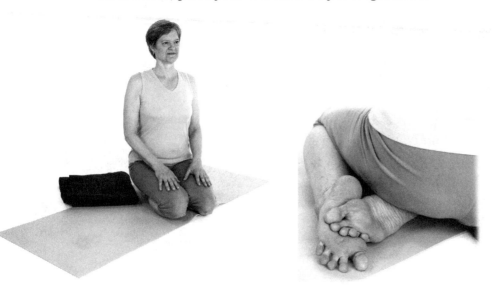

7. Deepen the twist with a wrapping action that begins behind the back of your left ribs and moves to the right.
8. Continue in the pose with rhythmic breathing: inhale, lift up the spine, and turn more as you exhale.
9. Level your shoulders; preserve a quiet face as you turn. Soften your diaphragm while maintaining strength in the arms and legs. Move farther with each exhalation.
10. Inhale as you return to center. Repeat on the other side.

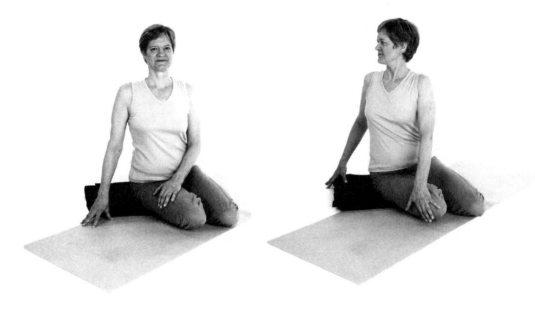

5. ARDHA MATSYENDRASANA

This seated twist is dedicated to Matsyendra, a fisherman thought to be the originator of Hatha Yoga. The literal translation of *matsyendra* is "Lord of the Fishes."

Purpose: To increase lateral rotation range and stretch the outer hips.

Contraindications: Absolute: pregnancy. Relative: total hip replacement, colostomy, herniated disc, vertebral fracture.

Props: A yoga mat and a blanket.

Avoiding pitfalls: Lengthen the spine upward to free it and the rib cage for rotation. Root down through the pelvic bones. Use your abdominal muscles to help you twist.

INSTRUCTIONS:

1. Sit on the edge of a folded blanket.
2. Fold your left leg so that the knee faces straight forward, and the foot rests outside your right hip.
3. Manually widen your buttocks and upper thighs.
4. Cross your right leg over your left, placing the right foot flat on the floor outside the left knee, with the right shin vertical.
5. Lift your spine as you inhale. Root down through both pelvic bones.
6. Exhale and turn to the right. Hold your right knee with your left hand; place your right hand behind you on the floor.
7. If you can twist more deeply, position the left elbow outside the right knee, pointing your left hand up.
8. Press your right leg and left arm firmly against each other, creating the power for a deep twist. Retain a long, vertical spine.
9. Continue the twist by wrapping the back of your left ribs to the right.
10. When the spine has revolved as far as possible, keep turning your inner body. Lift your spine farther with each inhalation; revolve somewhat farther as you exhale.
11. Release and repeat on the other side.

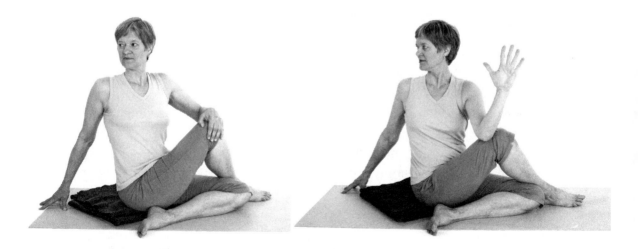

6. TRIANG MUKHAIKAPADA PASCHIMOTTANASANA (Trifold Forward Bend)

Purpose: To stretch the lower back, hips, thighs, and pelvis.

Contraindications: Knee restrictions, colostomy, total hip replacement.

Props: A yoga mat, a blanket or two, a belt, and a washcloth.

Avoiding pitfalls: Use enough lift under your hips to prevent knee pain in the bent leg.

INSTRUCTIONS:

1. Sit on the edge of a blanket folded to the width of your hips.
2. Fold your right foot back beside your right hip, toes going straight back with your ankle near your thigh. Extend your toes, especially the fourth and fifth ones, on both feet.
3. If your right ankle is stiff, put a folded washcloth under the ankle.
4. Manually pull your sitting bones and buttocks back and apart.
5. If you are leaning to the left, place another blanket under your left hip. This will lower your right hip relative to it.
6. Loop the belt around your left foot and hold both ends with your right hand. Placing your left hand on the floor at your side will help you to align your torso straight forward.

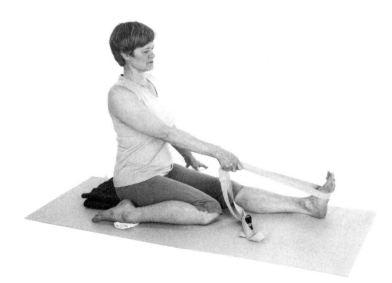

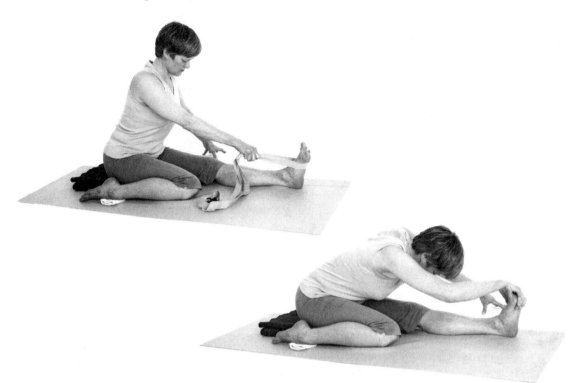

7. Inhaling, lift up through your spine, pulling the middle of your back in and up and your arms back in the shoulder joints.
8. Exhaling, bend forward from your hips, with your abdomen lifting up and your torso moving out over the left leg.
9. Hold your foot if you can reach it, and release your head down.
10. Maintain the pose for several breaths, keeping your legs active but softening and releasing in the upper body.

Forward bends remind one to bring awareness inside and become quiet.

---

7. PASCHIMOTTANASANA
(Full Stretch of the West Side of the Body)

Purpose: To stretch the back and the legs, to conclude a practice with a quiet mind.

Contraindications: Hamstring sprain, ischial bursitis.

Props: Two folded blankets and one belt.

Avoiding pitfalls: Make sure to straighten your legs fully, pressing your thighs down.

INSTRUCTIONS:

1. Sit on the edge of one folded blanket, with your legs extended forward and a belt looped around your feet.
2. Manually pull your sitting bones and thighs back and apart. This will help you tilt your pelvis forward.
3. Hug the leg muscles to the bones and stretch out through your feet, with your toes and kneecaps pointing straight up.
4. Place the other folded blanket on your legs if needed, to rest your head on later.
5. Firm your abdominal muscles and lift your spine up from the core of the pelvis.
6. Pull on the belt to connect your arms into the shoulders and to prepare to bend forward.
7. Prepare yourself for an extreme stretch as you inhale deeply.
8. Exhale, bend forward, and pull on the belt or reach to catch your feet.

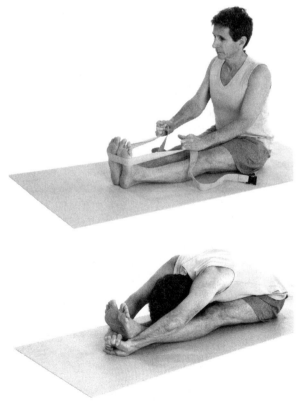

9. Extend forward evenly on the sides, front, and back of your torso.
10. Rest your head on the blanket or your legs and stay in the pose for a minute or so, breathing smoothly.
11. Soften your neck, shoulders, and upper back, but activate your quadriceps, pressing the backs of your knees down.
12. Attend to an inner stillness as you breathe smoothly.
13. When you are ready, come up softly to sit tall again and release.

Lumbar Spine *Asana*: Types of Action and Intensity

Name	Flexion	Extension	Lateral Bend	Twist	Strengthen Flexion	Strengthen Extension	Pelvic-Lumbar Coordination
■ BEGINNING							
*Windshield Wiper				1			2
Cat-Cow	2	2					1
Side Child's Pose	2		2				
*Child's Pose	2						
*Plank, Stage III					2	2	1
*Bhujangasana		2				2	2
*Salabhasana		2				3	1
*Adho Mukha Svanasana, Stage II: Wall Dog		1				2	3
*Standing Lunge with Wall		2				1	3
Standing Crescent			2				1
*Pressure Cooker		1					
*Chair Twist				3			1
Chair Malasana	3						
*Setu Bandhasana		2					1
*Supta Padangusthasana		1				2	2
■ INTERMEDIATE							
*Standing Lunge with Chair		2				1	3
*Utthita Trikonasana				1		1	2
*Utthita Parsvakonasana				2		1	2
Parivrtta Parsvakonasana				3		2	2
Uttanasana	3						
Ardha Bhekasana		2				2	1
Ustrasana with Chair		2				2	1
Parighasana with Chair			3			1	
Pigeon Pose with Bolster and Chair		3				2	2
*Janu Sirsasana	3			1			1
*Child's Pose	2						1

Name	Flexion	Extension	Lateral Bend	Twist	Strengthen Flexion	Strengthen Extension	Pelvic-Lumbar Coordination
■ CHALLENGING							
Viparita Dandasana Prep		2			1 (in and out)		2
Supta Virasana		2					1
Parivrtta Janu Sirsasana			3	3		1	2
Bharadvajasana		1		2		1	2
Ardha Matsyendrasana		1		2		1	3
Triang Mukhaikapada Paschimottanasana	2				1	1	
Paschimottanasana	3					1	

Note: Higher numbers indicate greater intensity.

CHAPTER 9

The Cervical Spine

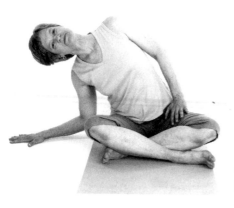

It is always rush hour in the neck. The strongest (and most important) reflexes function side by side with the ultimate of human volition: every bite, every breath, almost every movement and sensation, and each spoken word involves passage of impulses through the neck. In addition to housing the most autonomic and the most voluntary aspects of human life, the neck must be supple and versatile enough to turn in every direction as quickly and effortlessly as possible. The vertebrae are smaller and finer, yet a major artery, the vertebral artery, weaves into and out of them on its way to the brain.

Osteoarthritis erodes the integrity, distorts the fine angles, truncates the delicate fits, and mars the supple symmetry of the cervical spine. Turning your head creates a noise and brings an uncomfortable strain, and your shoulders tend to swivel along with your eyes to compensate. Sometimes your neck aches without any apparent cause, and lying down, instead of giving rest, may produce a sharp twinge.

At times, osteoarthritis narrows the cervical neuroforamina, the openings between the vertebrae through which nerve roots pass from the spine to the arms, hands, and viscera. Then there may be pain, numbness, paresthesias, and weakness in one or both upper limbs—in dramatic cases, weakness to the point of near paralysis. Since the neck is such a compact and dynamic region, even swallowing can be impaired.

As if this were not enough, the shoulders and arms are held up by connections with the head and neck, placing the full weight of anything lifted by the arms on the cervical vertebrae. And though all this weight bearing might tend to make the muscles taut and solid, such tightness can compromise the nerves of the brachial plexus.

In addition to pinching nerves, the main effect of arthritis in the neck is limited range of motion. This is particularly obvious with rotation, a motion that is so vital to everyday activities. In what follows we not only address cervical range of motion directly but also offer some poses that integrate thoracic and cervical motion, coordinate their movements to maximize twist, and divide up the strain of shearing forces.

Yoga can do little to reduce swelling in the neuroforamina. But yoga can reduce compression of nerve roots and even alleviate swallowing disorders. Yoga can accomplish this in four ways: (1) by improving the suppleness of the muscles, (2) by increasing the versatility of the joints, (3) by refining the coordination of the various muscle groups in the neck and adjoining regions of the shoulder and thoracic spine, and (4) by facilitating relaxation. In this way yoga can help in handling the seemingly contradictory tasks of increasing strength and flexibility, adding the soothing element of calm to maximize the balance between them.

There are two common misalignments of the neck (see Figure 9 on next page), which we call the "tucker" (the head pulled back, neck too straight) and the "thruster" (head pushed forward, neck curved improperly). Both cause excessive strain in the muscles and joints of the neck. Both become habitual, and therefore might seem "normal." As you consider your own neck alignment, please be open to trying something new, even if it feels odd at first.

Four Anusara Yoga actions provide a valuable template for realigning the neck and balancing strength with flexibility.

- *Inner Body Bright*—The inside of the chest swells and lifts in the front, sides, and back. Taking a deep breath is one good way to feel this action, which readies you for what is to come.

- Move the top of the throat back, raising the tone of the anterior muscles of the neck. This is especially important for thrusters.
- *Shoulder Loop*—The shoulder blades pull toward each other. This tone in the upper back prevents the upper spine from collapsing, and retracts your upper arms. Slide the shoulder blades slightly down the back, without losing the lift that you created as you took the deep breath (for Inner Body Bright). The Shoulder Loop also includes a lift of the chin, tilting the tops of the ears slightly back. This part of Shoulder Loop is important for tuckers because it reestablishes the natural lordotic curve of the cervical spine.
- Float the neck and head up, relaxing your ears. Imagine a string drawing the top of your head straight up, or an overhead set of earphones pulling you up taller. For thrusters, floating the *back* of the head up is important. This corresponds to the Skull Loop (see Appendix III). Once you have balanced your head right on top of the spine (see "Normal" in figure below), then the whole head can float up evenly. This creates a feeling of spacious lightness.

Before and after you perform the neck postures we are about to describe, check your neck alignment with a mirror or a friend. Your goal is for your ears to be over your shoulders when viewed from the side, and your nose to be centered over your sternum when viewed from the front.

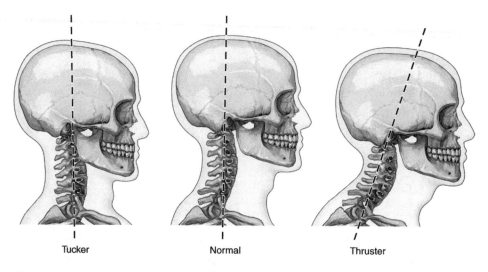

Tucker   Normal   Thruster

Figure 9. *Variants of cervical posture.*

Poses

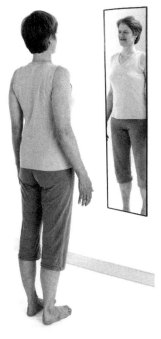

1. *TADASANA (Mountain Pose)—See page 59. Use a mirror to check your alignment.

2. COSMIC HEAD REST

Purpose: To strengthen the upper back and neck extensors and reinforce the natural arch of the neck with an isometric action.

Contraindications: Cervical vertebral instability, including spondylolisthesis, Chiari malformations.

Prop: A chair.

Avoiding pitfalls: Keep all sides of your neck long. Work diligently; do not overwork.

INSTRUCTIONS

1. Sit in a chair and adjust your thighs back and apart, as in Pressure Cooker (see page 73). This will help you to sit tall. Interlace your fingers behind your head.

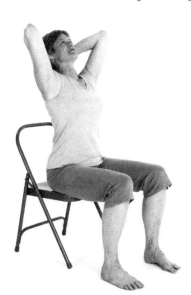

2. Keeping your upper back firm, tilt your head backward into your hands. Look up at a comfortable angle.
3. Balance these two goals:
   - Move back through the sides of your upper neck and ears.
   - Keep the front throat open and long.
4. Stretch up through the crown of your head. Root down through your pelvis and legs.
5. Do not forget to breathe while you hold the pose!
6. Return to center and release your hands down.

3. THE THINKER (Viparita [reverse] Cosmic Head Rest)

Purpose: To strengthen the neck flexors, which will help to free the extensors and prevent unnecessary compression.

Contraindication: Cervical vertebral instability.

Props: A chair and a table.

Avoiding pitfalls: Do not collapse the upper back. Keep your shoulders back.

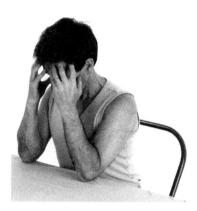

INSTRUCTIONS:

1. Sit tall, shoulders back. Rest your elbows on the table.
2. Inhale and lengthen your neck and head up.
3. Exhale and bend your head forward just a little; press your forehead into your hands.
4. Continue for a few breaths, then bring your head up.

4. *CHAIR TWIST—See page 75.

5. CHAIR MALASANA (Seated Partial Inversion)

Purpose: To give traction to the cervical spine.

Contraindications: Cerebrovascular disease, wet macular degeneration, history of vasovagal episodes.

Prop: A chair.

Avoiding pitfalls: Extend forward maximally through the whole upper body to give the best angle for the neck.

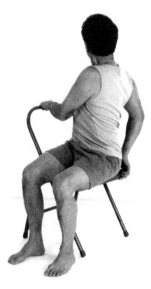

Twisting the entire spine helps to coordinate the different segments of the spine: the thoracic vertebrae take on some of the rotation when you turn your head.

INSTRUCTIONS:

1. Sit on the front edge of your chair with your legs wide apart.

2. Manually pull your buttocks back and apart, which will free you to tilt your pelvis forward.

3. Inhale; lift up your spine and chest.

4. Exhale and bend forward. Fold your torso between your legs.

5. Rest your hands on the floor. Hang your head straight down.

6. Lightly retract your upper arms into the shoulders, then stretch your arms forward. Maintain that action as you continue to release your neck down.

7. To exit the pose, extend your head and chest forward, support yourself with elbows on thighs, inhale, and swing up.

6. SHOULDERS BACK HEAD FORWARD

Purpose: To stretch the neck extensors while keeping the shoulders back.

Contraindications: Herniated cervical disc, rotator cuff syndrome.

Prop: A belt.

Avoiding pitfalls: Keep your upper back erect but not rigid. Avoid overly tightening your front neck muscles. Avoid over-arching your lower back.

INSTRUCTIONS:

1. Stand with the belt looped around your wrists with your arms behind you.

2. Inhale and lift your inner body up, making the sides of your body very long.

3. Firm your shoulder blades onto your back to support this tall posture. Pull your upper arms back.

4. Press your arms out against the belt.

5. Inhale again; lengthen up through your neck.

6. Exhaling, move your head forward and down toward your chest until you feel a good pull on the back of your neck.

7. Stay for several breaths, then inhale and raise your head.

8. Release your arms from the belt.

7. "ACHA"

This pose imitates the Indian tilting head movement that means "okay."

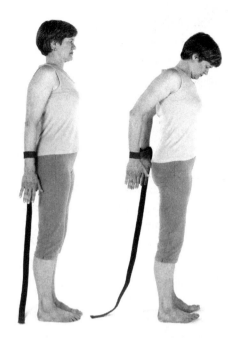

Purpose: To improve sideward tilt of the neck without thoracic movement.

Contraindications: Chiari malformations, cervical vertebral instability, inner ear dysfunction.

Prop: A belt.

Avoiding pitfalls: Your head will tend to bend forward. A little of that is okay, but try to align your head with your shoulder as you tilt. Retain a vertical upper back.

INSTRUCTIONS:

1. Stand tall. Hang a belt over your right shoulder. Hold the ends with your right hand.

2. Inhale. Lift your inner body up. (Remember the action described before: Inner Body Bright.)

3. Firm your shoulder blades onto your back to support this tall posture.

4. Inhale again and softly lengthen up through your neck. Lift the front and back equally.

5. Exhaling, tilt your head to the left side.

6. Pull on the belt with your right hand to isolate the stretch in your neck.

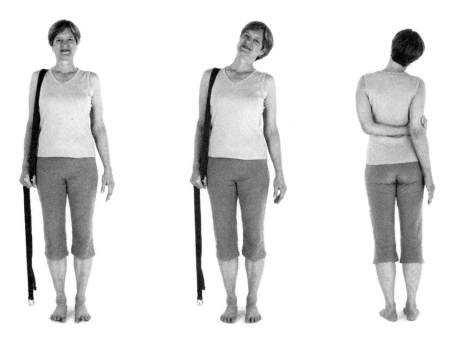

7. Hold this for a few seconds, then return to center and repeat on the other side.

8. For greater intensity, reach behind and catch the arm on the side to which your head is tilting, to keep the shoulders horizontal.

---

8. *PRASARITA PADOTTANASANA WITH BENT KNEES

Purpose: To improve traction and rotation of cervical spine, also to stretch the hips.

Contraindication: Poor balance.

Props: A yoga mat and possibly two blocks.

Avoiding pitfalls: Widen your thighs as you bend your legs. The leg muscles stay active.

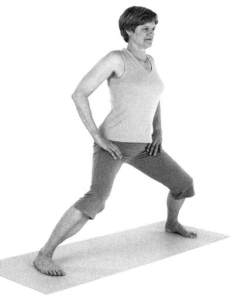

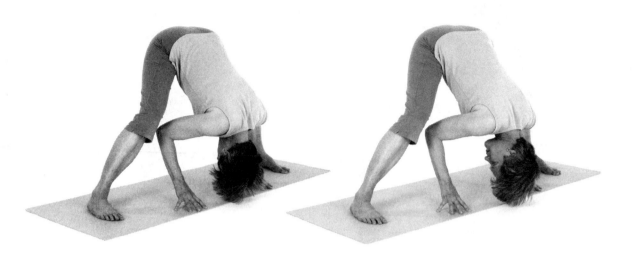

INSTRUCTIONS:

1. Place your legs wide apart and parallel. Bring your hands to your hips.
2. Bend your knees and lift up through your spine as you inhale.
3. Exhale and bend forward, tilting from the hips as much as possible.
4. Touch the floor or blocks lightly with your hands.
5. Pull your arms up into the shoulder sockets, but let your head hang loosely down.
6. Move your head and neck cautiously in all directions—nodding your head yes, turning side to side, and shaking your head no.
7. Let your head hang again in center for a few breaths, releasing down.
8. Step your feet closer together. Root down through your legs, stretch your chest and head forward, place your hands on your hips, and come up with a strong inhalation.

---

9. SLOW METRONOME (Sitting Spinal Tilt)

Purpose: To coordinate neck and lateral thoracic spine movements.

Contraindications: Ankylosing spondylitis with fusion, thoracic vertebral fracture, severe degenerative scoliosis.

Props: A yoga mat, possibly a blanket.

Avoiding pitfalls: Retain your shoulder blades firmly together on your back in the Shoulder Loop; avoid leaning forward.

INSTRUCTIONS:

1. Sit cross-legged on the floor. If your knees are higher than your hips, sit up on a folded blanket or pad.
2. Inhale; lift up through your whole spine and torso (Inner Body Bright).
3. Pull your shoulder blades toward the spine and slightly down, lifting the front of your chest up.
4. Exhale and lean to the right as you rest your right hand on the floor beside you and your left hand on your hip or thigh. Make an even curved shape from your left hip to the top of your head. Soften inside.
5. Inhale. Return to vertical.
6. Exhale and bend to the left side as you place your left palm on the floor beside you.
7. Repeat as above several more times to each side. Movements should be as fluid and naturally expressive as possible. Accept whatever range is comfortable for you.

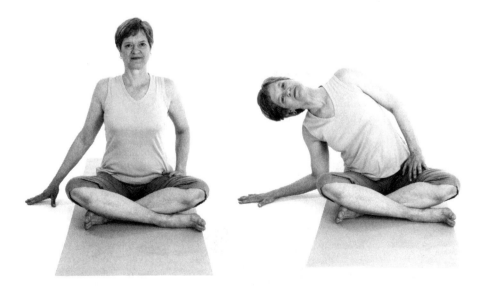

10. *BHUJANGASANA—See page 89.

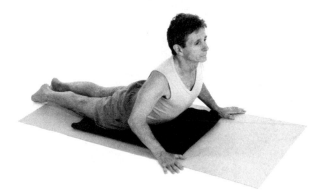

This back bend increases extension and encourages better posture. It also strengthens the neck and upper back.

11. *JATHARA PARIVARTANASANA—See page 84.

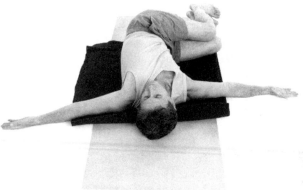

This spinal twist will help to coordinate the different segments of the spine.

12. *SETU BANDHASANA—See page 81.

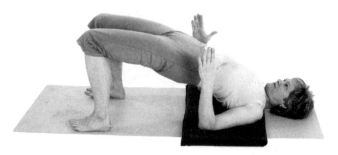

This back bend stretches the neck, encourages better posture, and strengthens the upper back.

13. MOUNTAIN BROOK

Purpose: To support in a resting position the natural curves of the spine.

Contraindications: None.

Props: A yoga mat, a bolster, and two blankets.

Avoiding pitfalls: Take the time to set up the props so you are comfortable.

INSTRUCTIONS:

1. Fold one blanket into a long rectangle and place it on your mat where your upper chest will be when you lie down on your back.
2. Leaving a space for your shoulders to rest, place another blanket down toward the top of your mat. Make a long roll with the side of it to provide support for your neck. What is left after making this roll will pad your head on the floor. The size of the roll should be determined by level of comfort under the curve of your neck. Place the bolster across the mat where your knees will be.
3. Lie down on your back, with the bolster under your knees and the folded blanket under the back of your chest. The bottom of your shoulder blades should be supported by the distant edge of the blanket nearer the bolster.
4. Adjust the other blanket to fit snugly under your neck. It should support the natural arch there.
5. Extend your arms out at a comfortable angle from your sides, palms up.
6. Relax and breathe deeply.

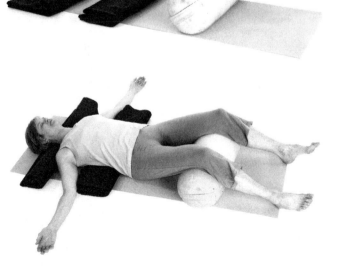

7. If any part of your body is uncomfortable, roll to the side, sit up, and adjust the props.

8. Stay in the position for five to fifteen minutes. Enjoy the support of the props and the heaviness of your body.

9. When you are ready to get up, roll to the side and slowly sit up.

Restorative poses like this give the contours of the body full support and allow you to stay in the position longer, relaxing all joints and muscles deeply.

Cervical *Asana*: Types of Action and Intensity

Name	Lateral Rotation	Lateral Flexion	Flexion	Extension	Traction	Rest
*Tadasana (with mirror)						1
Cosmic Head Rest				2		
The Thinker			2			
*Chair Twist	2					
Chair Malasana			2		2	1
Shoulders Back Head Forward			2			
"Acha"		2				
*Prasarita Padottanasana with Bent Knees			1		2	
Slow Metronome		2				
*Bhujangasana				2		
*Jathara Parivartanasana	1					
*Setu Bandhasana			2			
Mountain Brook				1		3

Note: Poses are graded for the intensity with which they engage the effects listed at the top of the columns: 1 = moderate degree; 2 = substantial degree; 3 = near maximal.

CHAPTER 10

The Knees

The knees are the largest joints in the body. This fact in itself prompts some to rank them among the most vulnerable to injury. They also bear a great deal of weight, loading and unloading with every step, every time one gets up, and on every stair. Further, unlike the hips they move only in a single plane, without very much adaptability to linear or rotating pressures from the side. We can protect the hips when we fall by bending our knees. But what do we have to cushion the knees? Only the ankles and feet, with their much more limited size, strength, and ranges of motion.

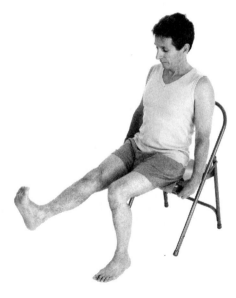

Unlike most joints, there are three bones participating in the knee joint (see Figure 1 on page 25). The kneecap or patella is a sesamoid bone, a bone enclosed in a tendon. This gives additional leverage to the quadriceps in extending the knees, very much like putting a block beneath a hammer's head when pulling out a nail. But the patella is also exposed to the trauma that comes naturally to all bipeds.

If you could examine the underside of the patella closely, you would find a wonderfully precise structure, like a well-cut, many-faceted jewel. The thigh bone, or femur, ends at the knee in the form of two egg-sized half ellipses side by side. The two shapes are unequal in size. Therefore, the joint's center of rotation moves with each infinitesimal change of angle as it goes from flexed to extended. The underside of the patella interfaces with the tibia and the femur in an ever-changing spatial and mechanical relationship. So we have a very delicate, vulnerable structure exposed to near-constant trauma. Even minimal swelling upsets the balance. Any imbalance leads to regions of exaggerated stress. As we have seen several times already, this is the formula for osteoarthritis.

But the picture is broader and deeper. The knee has its own internal shock absorbers, the medial and lateral menisci: a thick figure-of-eight-shaped cartilage that sits on top of the flat joint surface of the tibia, and cradles the elliptical hemispheres of the femur. This too can be worn down and injured. Generally the medial meniscus is affected before and more seriously than the lateral one.

How do we resist or at least minimize this wearing down? As you will recall from Chapter 3, joint health is primarily maintained by the circulation of the joint fluid, an excellent viscous lubricant that provides the oxygen and proteins needed for joint repair, and carries away the waste products of metabolism. Yoga, by moving the joint to the extremes of motion (but not farther), helps this process considerably.

Because the knee is so much affected by movements in its neighboring joints (especially the hip, sacroiliac, lumbar spine, and ankle) the yoga we offer for those areas can protect the knee a great deal. Flexibility in the hips means less demand on the knees. Strength in the lumbar spine and abdominal musculature reduces the load on the knees, and as stated, flexibility in the ankles cushions the impact that the knees might otherwise absorb. So if the knees are your area of concern, please practice the poses from the chapters on these other joints as well as those in this one.

Two pairs of opposite actions serve to stabilize and align the knee for safety in all types of movements and positions. First, let us look at the alignment of the knee in the frontal plane. In many people, the lower legs bow outward, and the knees and thighs angle in toward the midline. Often the arches of the feet are collapsed as well. What is needed for better alignment is to balance the weight on the four corners of the feet (see page 235), to bring the shins in toward the midline, and to widen the thighs, until each leg lines up in one plumb line from ankle to hip joint. This Shins-In-Thighs-Out action is exemplified by the Pressure Cooker (see page 73). Shins-In-Thighs-Out aligns the kneecaps to point straight forward toward the second toes. This is also called tracking the knee, and you can check it for yourself in a mirror.

The second alignment to consider is the forward-back relationship of the lower and upper leg, as observed from the side. Knees that are hyperextended push back too far, reducing stability and distributing pressure unevenly inside the joint. The Shin Loop and the Thigh Loop (see Appendix III) comprise an excellent safeguard. Pressing the ball of the foot down while standing advances the top of the shin bone forward, and then flexing the quadriceps fixes the femur without overextending the knee. These actions may seem complex at first, but with practice they can be incorporated into many poses. You will recognize them in the instructions below.

Poses

1. CHAIR HEEL SLIDE

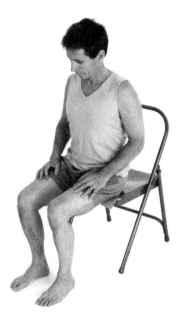

Purpose: To track the alignment of the knee, coordinate knee, ankle, foot, and thigh movements made during normal walking, and gently strengthen the quadriceps, all with minimal weight bearing.

Contraindication: Recent abdominal surgery.

Prop: A chair.

Avoiding pitfalls: Watch and move carefully, coordinating the movement between all the anatomical components. Do not lift the straight-legged knee above the bent knee at any time.

INSTRUCTIONS:

1. Sit on the edge of a chair with feet flat on the floor and knees bent ninety degrees. The thighs are parallel and at the same level.

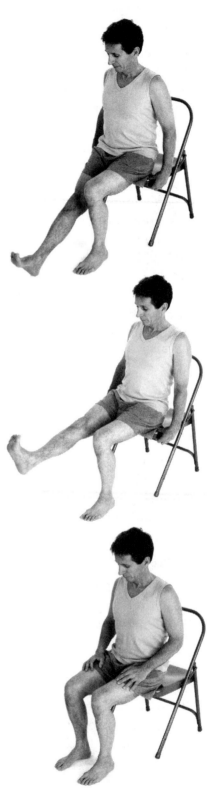

2. Slide the right heel outward along the floor until the right knee is fully extended. At this point the right thigh slants downward away from the left thigh.

3. After sliding the right leg out until the knee is straight, lift the entire right leg until the right thigh is parallel with the left.

4. Maintain parallel thighs while bending the right knee and returning the right foot to its place beside the left.

5. Repeat five to ten times.

6. Repeat with the left leg.

7. To reduce the intensity, from the initial sitting position, slide the right heel out about halfway. The knee will not straighten fully. Raise the right thigh until it is parallel to the left, even though the knee is still somewhat bent. Lower the foot back directly under the knee, keeping the thighs parallel throughout the process. Repeat on the other side. This pose can gradually metamorphose into the more intense version by gradually increasing the distance you slide the heel until the knee is straight.

Both versions of this action pose are gentle but require precision and full attention. Coordination and proprioception at ankle, knee, and hip are improved significantly, all of which are critical to knee care.

2. *PRESSURE COOKER—
See page 73.

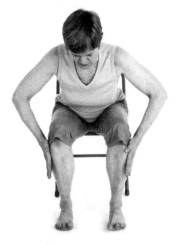

This pose uses an isometric action in the legs to realign the sacroiliac joint, hips, and knees.

3. *STANDING LUNGE WITH
CHAIR—See page 72.

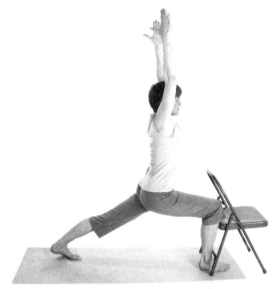

You can practice tracking the front knee carefully in this pose while also stretching the calf and hip of your back leg.

4. *LOTUS PREP WITH
WALL—See page 78.

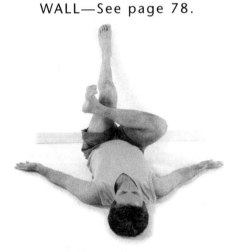

This deep hip stretch helps take pressure off the knee.

5. *SETU BANDHASANA—
See page 81.

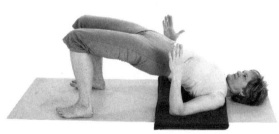

Thigh muscles are strengthened in this pose.

6. *SUPTA PADANGUSTHASANA—See page 83.

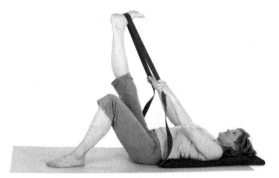

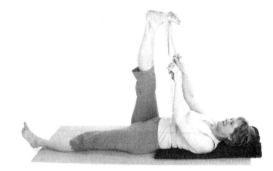

This excellent overall leg stretch helps straighten knees with the hips flexed.

Tight hamstring muscles strain the lower back.

7. *JANU SIRSASANA— See page 91.

8. *WALL QUAD— See page 76.

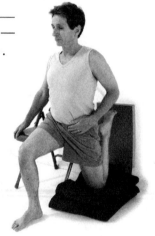

This seated leg stretch also benefits the hips and spine.

This is a deep stretch of the quadriceps.

9. *ADHO MUKHA SVANASANA— See page 62.

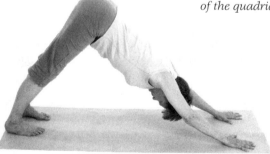

You can see your knees in this pose. Practice aligning them carefully.

10. UTKATASANA (Chair Pose, two stages)

Purpose: To align and strengthen the quadriceps, adductors, and abductors, and to coordinate knees, hips, ankles, and lumbar spine.

Contraindications: Imbalance, acromioclavicular subluxation, rotator cuff tear, severe osteoporosis, profound weakness, moderate or severe anterior cruciate tear, chondromalacia patellae.

Prop: A wall.

Avoiding pitfalls: Take care to align the knees to track the kneecaps straight forward over the second toes, and to align the lower back—neither too arched nor too curved.

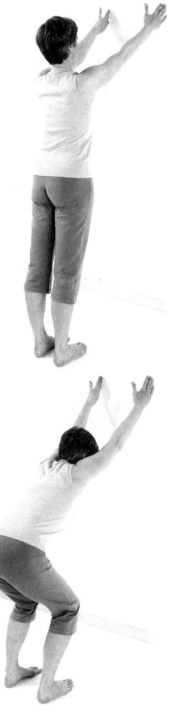

INSTRUCTIONS:

Stage I

1. Stand a few feet from a wall, facing it.
2. Reach your arms forward, shoulder-width apart, and touch your fingertips lightly on the wall, just above eye level.
3. Set your arms deeply into the shoulder sockets. Stretch your legs and strongly draw your abdomen in toward your core.
4. Lift your toes and root the four corners of your feet down (see page 235 for foot illustration).
5. Inhale, extend your upper body up from the inside, and arch your lower back slightly.
6. Exhale, bend your knees, and reach your hips back. Make one long line from fingers to hips.
7. Widen your thighs apart, as in Pressure Cooker (see page 73), without widening the lower legs. Your arms will lean more firmly on the wall.
8. Curl your tailbone down and lift your lower abdomen. This will support your lower back

and lessen the arch there. Take special care to track the kneecaps straight forward.

9. Splay the toes apart. Press the balls of the feet and the heels down.
10. Breathe strongly to energize the pose.
11. Inhale as you return to standing.

This pose brings tremendous inner and outer strength.

Stage II

1. Stand facing away from a wall, and adjust the distance so that when you bend your knees and hips, your hips will rest against the wall. Set your feet hip-distance apart and parallel.
2. Inhaling, bend your knees, reach your hips back to the wall, and raise your arms to the sides in one vigorous movement.
3. Stretch your toes, especially the fourth and fifth ones, and root the heels down.
4. Re-create the widening of the thighs as in Pressure Cooker (see page 73), tracking the kneecaps straight forward over the second and third toes.
5. As your hips draw back, allow the lower back to arch, producing a deep fold in your hips.
6. Lift the lower abdomen up to support the lower back and lessen the lumbar curve.
7. Breathe calmly and maintain the position for as long as you can.
8. Come back up and lower your arms.

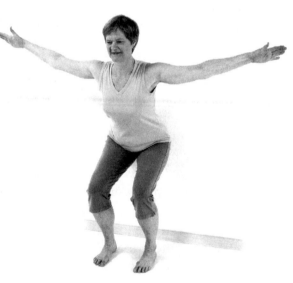

11. *UTTHITA PARSVAKONASANA—See page 67.

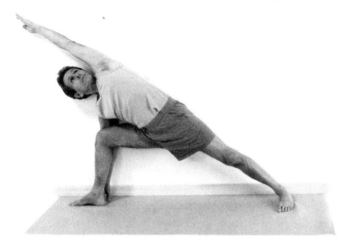

This vigorous standing pose stretches and strengthens the knees.

12. UTTANASANA (Standing Forward Bend)

Purpose: To stretch the thoracic spine and the legs.

Contraindications: Herniated nucleus pulposus, imbalance.

Props: A yoga mat, two blocks if your legs are stiff.

Avoiding pitfalls: Keep your leg muscles working, whether your knees are bent or straight. Avoid letting the knees fall in toward the midline. Let your head release. Come out of the pose smoothly to avoid dizziness.

INSTRUCTIONS:

1. Stand with your feet hip-width apart.
2. Stretch your toes and lift them up, which activates the whole lower leg. Balance your weight on the four corners of your feet.
3. Retain the elevated toes, then squeeze your shins in toward the midline, and widen your thighs apart. You can lean forward a little to do this.
4. With thighs still wide, pull your tailbone down and your spine up vertically.

5. Inhale and stretch fully up from inside.
6. Exhale, bend forward, and touch the floor or two blocks. Bend your knees if necessary, taking care to track them straight forward.
7. Come down far enough to feel the pull on your hamstring muscles.
8. Retain your arms deep in their sockets, even as you reach down.
9. If you can straighten your knees and you want more intensity, hold your ankles and pull yourself farther down.
10. Avoid pushing your knees back; instead, press the balls of the feet down and lift up the quadriceps.
11. Balance your use of strength with an attitude of surrender and release. Breathe evenly.
12. To come up, bring your hands to your waist. Root down through your legs to the four corners of your feet, extend your head and chest forward, and lift up smoothly as you inhale.
13. Exhale and release your hands.

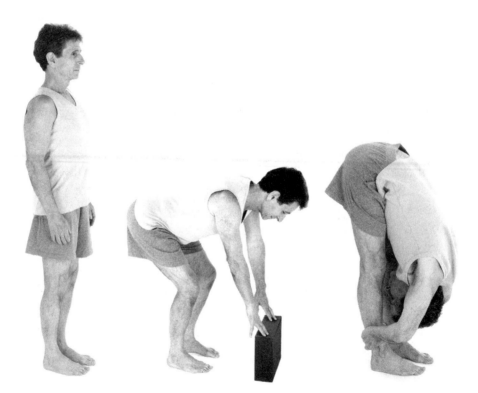

Knee *Asana*: Range of Motion and Degree of Strengthening

Name	ROM Flexion[a]	ROM Extension[a]	Strength Flexion	Strength Extension	Additional Benefits to Knee's Function
Chair Heel Slide	90	180		1	Coordinates hips, knee, ankles
*Pressure Cooker	90	90			Strengthens abductors[b]
*Standing Lunge with Chair	90	180	2	3	Strengthens vastus medialis and lateralis
*Lotus Prep with Wall	45	180			Stretches iliotibial band
*Setu Bandhasana	45	90		1	Extends hip joint
*Supta Padangusthasana	45	180			Flexes hip joint, stretches hamstrings
*Janu Sirsasana	35	180		2	Flexes hip joint, stretches hamstrings
*Wall Quad	20	90	2		Extends hip joint while flexing knee
*Adho Mukha Svanasana	180	180		2	Strengthens vastus medialis, refines weight bearing
Utkatasana	135	180		3	Coordinates hips, knee, ankles with torso
*Utthita Parsvakonasana	90	180	2	2	Coordinates hip external rotation with flexion and extension
Uttanasana	180	180		2	Challenges balance and improves hip flexion

Note: ROM = range of motion (in degrees) always measuring 180 degrees as a straightened knee. These are maximal amounts in the correct pose, not what is required to try. Degree of strengthening is denoted by ascending numbers: 1 = moderate; 2 = substantial; 3 = near maximal.

[a]In all measurements the straight leg is 180 degrees.

[b]With the actions known as Muscular Energy and Inner Spiral the adductors are active here as well.

CHAPTER 11

The Sacroiliac Joints

Sacroiliitis is perhaps the most underdiagnosed of all the conditions that afflict the back. Many physicians still believe that healthy sacroiliac joints do not move, so they find nothing pathological about a fused

sacroiliac joint in Reiter's syndrome, psoriatic arthritis, ankylosing spondylitis, or gout. In truth, the keystone-shaped sacrum is composed of bones that fused together early in life, but the sacrum itself does indeed move *relative to the iliac crests* (see Figure 10b on page 196). In fact, the sacrum is analogous to the universal gear in an automobile. It mediates between the lower body and the upper body, doing all it can to keep the body erect and hold it steady over moving legs, often while the upper body is bent and contorting to move and manipulate

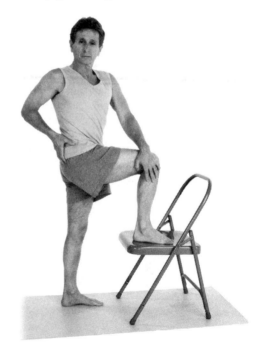

objects, or to do the numberless things that fill a busy day and night. Think of the different roles the upper and lower body play in lifting a suitcase, dressing, getting into the backseat of a taxi, typing, examining a patient, swinging a tennis racquet, and dancing. The sacroiliac joint does its mediating job in all of these activities.

If you look at a human skeleton, you will see a striking characteristic of the sacroiliac joint: Unlike the horizontal planes of the tibial plateau at the knee, or the ankle bones at that mortise, or even the curving top of the hip's socket, the sacroiliac joint is a *vertical* joint. What kind of way is that to hold something up? If you want to place down a tea tray or a napkin, you would use the horizontal surface of a tabletop long before attempting to put it on the table's vertical leg! The large, three-dimensional sacroiliac joint may be that way because humanoids used to walk on all fours (rendering the joint horizontal), and the structure hasn't evolved to reflect our upright posture. Or perhaps this orientation and shape really are most effective for the joint's delicate balancing act between the supportive role below and the flexibility demanded by the actions of the structures above it. In any event, the joint has adapted by developing very powerful ligaments that crisscross from the sacrum to the iliac bones and back again, and stalagmites and stalactites that interdigitate and hold the parts together.

If the heart is the center of the circulatory system, the sacrum is the heart of the musculoskeletal system. It bears the brunt of all our weight and is the vertex of all movement where balance in space is a factor. This goes for climbing stairs, swimming, sexual activity, and taking a book from a library shelf.

Is it so strange that many older people have trouble moving because of pain in this region? The same powerful forces that hold the functioning joint together are formidable adversaries when it comes to correcting a joint that is out of kilter. Considerable leverage must be generated to overcome the ligaments that then hold the joints tightly in the *wrong* alignment. Like the knee, the sacrum is unable to share or alternate the constant stress it is subject to, and an ill-fitting joint on one side definitely constrains adaptation on the other. If ever there were primary victims of wear and tear, it is these saddle-shaped sacroiliac joints. For these reasons we give them a lot of attention.

One aspect of the yoga strategy that we use here promotes movement to prevent the formation and crystallization of fibrils and collagen,

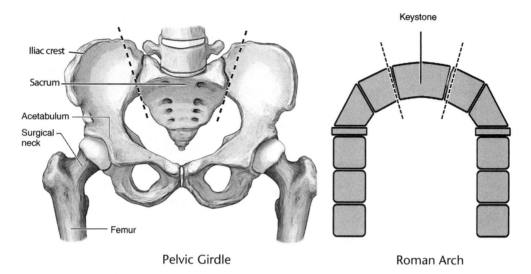

Pelvic Girdle   Roman Arch

Figure 10a. *As the keystone of a Roman arch is held up by gravity's downward pull, the sacrum is suspended between symmetrical forces of sufficient magnitude to keep the spine aloft.*

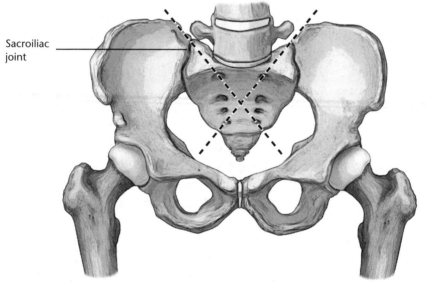

Axes of Nutation

Figure 10b. *The forces and geometry of the sacrum cause small but crucial movements of the sacrum along diagonal axes, called nutation.*

which will bind the joints together. Adhesions like these threaten joint mobility but they can be stretched and ultimately broken to free the joint. However, one must begin early. Because these conditions are frequently hereditary, one has some warning of their impending appearance and therefore can prepare and work to stave off the consequences of the legacy early in the game.

Another cause of sacroiliac pain is instability, when the joint is too loose and too mobile rather than tightly bound. However, this occurs rarely with osteoarthritis. Although there are some stabilizing poses in what follows, we focus on increasing sacroiliac movement. If you believe that too much motion is your problem, please consult a physiatrist, osteopath, or physical therapist before embarking on these poses.

The Anusara Yoga principles, consistent with Mr. Iyengar's methods, that we find helpful in the sacroiliac area are as follows:

- *Foundation*—Set your feet carefully. Placing the feet parallel will allow for proper spacing in the joint, whereas a turned-out stance can compress it.
- *Muscular Energy*—An unstable sacroiliac joint is extremely painful. Proper coordination of the muscles in the pelvis will help to stabilize the sacroiliac joints.
- *Inner Spiral*—Turn the thighs in, move them back, and widen them apart. These actions provide lateral space in the joint, and are balanced by Outer Spiral and Organic Energy, described below.
- *Outer Spiral*—Pull the tailbone down and revolve the thighs out enough for the knees to face forward without losing the width from Inner Spiral.
- *Organic Energy*—From the Focal Point at the base of the sacrum, stretch down through the legs and simultaneously up through the spine. This action provides vertical space in these saddle-shaped joints.

You will find symmetrical and asymmetrical poses interspersed here. The asymmetrical ones are more challenging and opening, the symmetrical ones more stabilizing, neutralizing, and strengthening. Try them all, and then focus on the ones that do what you need.

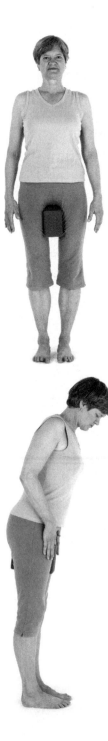

Poses

1. TADASANA WITH BLOCK
(variation of Mountain Pose)

Purpose: To provide space and stability in the sacroiliac area.

Contraindication: Total hip replacement.

Props: A yoga mat and a block.

Avoiding pitfalls: Stay aware and work patiently.

INSTRUCTIONS:

1. Place your feet hip width apart and parallel. Place a block between your upper thighs.
2. Adjust your stance so that you can root the four corners of each foot into the floor (the big toe mound will tend to lift up). (This is Foundation.)
3. Lift your toes up to engage the muscular strength of your lower legs. Squeeze the shins in toward the midline. (This is Muscular Energy.)
4. With the shins firm, squeeze the block with your thighs, then move it back. You can lean forward in your torso to make that easier to do. Make the tops of your thighs line up vertically over your ankles.
5. Widen your thighs laterally away from the block, as if to let it fall out. Avoid turning the knees in or out. Instead, widen the back and front of the thighs equally. (Instructions 4 and 5 comprise the Inner Spiral.)
6. Retain that width and the retracted position of your thighs as you pull the tailbone down, lengthening your lower back. (This initiates

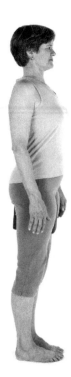

the Outer Spiral.) It may help to have one hand on your sacrum as it moves down and one hand on your abdomen as it lifts up. The thighs will tend to move forward and turn out as well, but the block gives you a clear reference point to help keep them back. Have your kneecaps pointing straight forward.

7. From the base of your sacrum, extend strongly down through your legs and pull up through your whole spine. (This is Organic Energy.)

8. Breathe and hold the pose for about thirty seconds, then release and remove the block.

2. *WINDSHIELD WIPER—See page 80.

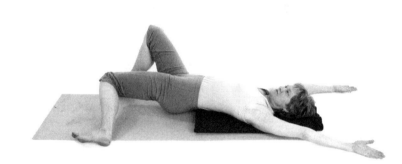

This pose helps to widen the back of the pelvis.

3. *LOTUS PREP WITH WALL—See page 78.

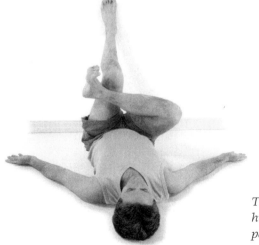

This pose safely stretches the deep hip muscles at the back of the pelvis that may restrict movement.

4. *SUPTA PADANGUSTHASANA—See page 83.

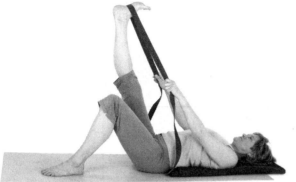 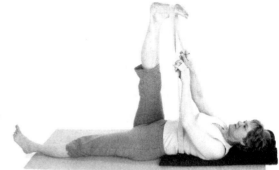

In this hamstring stretch you can practice working your legs strongly while stabilizing the pelvis.

Tight hamstring muscles strain the lower back by restricting knee-hip-sacroliac motion.

5. BHUJANGASANA (variation with shin belt)

Purpose: To strengthen the back and facilitate fuller use of the legs to provide space in the sacroiliac area.

Contraindications: Fused ankylosing spondylitis, Chiari malformations, bridging spondylitis, cervical spinal stenosis.

Props: A yoga mat, a blanket, and a belt.

Avoiding pitfalls: Belt your legs so they are about hip-width apart, not wider or narrower than that. Keep your shoulders back and do not overuse your arms. If you get up into the pose and find your shoulders around your ears and your chest collapsed, come down and start over. This pose is about expanding the inside of you, and supporting yourself with the muscles of your spine. The preparations are numerous but worth it!

INSTRUCTIONS:

1. Make a belt loop that will encircle your lower legs, to keep them hip-width apart. Put it on just below the knees, around the thicker part of your calves.

2. Lie on your stomach with a blanket spread beneath you for cushioning under your pelvis.

3. Lift one leg up an inch and pull it back. Repeat with the other leg. This is to keep a good length in the lower back.

4. Roll your legs so that the heels, thighs, and pelvis widen in the back, as you did in Tadasana with Block (page 198). Push out strongly enough to feel the restraint of the belt.

5. Pull your tailbone toward your heels and toward the floor. This is to stabilize your lower back so that you can stretch forward more strongly. The tailbone action will initiate an outward rotation down the legs: the heels and backs of the knees now face straight up.

6. Lift up onto your forearms briefly to pull your upper body away from your legs.

7. Lie back down and put your hands next to the sides of your chest, with your palms down, fingers pointing outward a bit, and forehead on the floor.

8. Lift your shoulders away from the floor, with your head still touching the floor and keeping your shoulders square across.

9. Inhale; lengthen forward through your whole torso. Expand from inside.

10. Contract your upper back muscles, and move the shoulder blades in toward the spine.

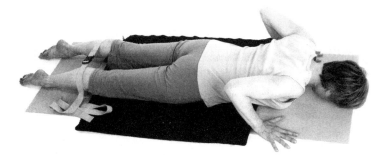

11. Now you are ready to lift up into the pose—curl up with your head and chest, keeping your shoulders back.

12. Press carefully down through your arms to lift more, but keep your arms bent and the upper arms and shoulders back.

13. Come up to the height that feels right to you, expanding forward

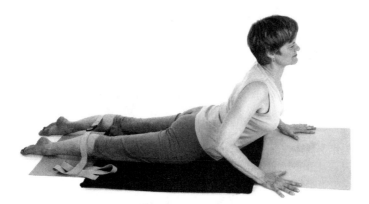

with freedom. Keep pushing the thighs apart into the resistance of the belt.

14. Stay up for several breaths, then soften and release down.

---

6. SUKHASANA
(Crossed-Leg Seated Pose with Knee Resistance)

Purpose: To integrate and protect the sacroiliac joint by bringing the thigh bones (femurs) deeper in the hip sockets and toning the lower back muscles as the sacrum and spine lift up.

Contraindication: Spondylolisthesis.

Prop: A blanket or two to sit on.

Avoiding pitfalls: Use enough support under your hips to enable you to sit with your whole spine erect, not slouched, with your knees lower than or level with the top of your pelvis.

INSTRUCTIONS:

1. Sit cross-legged on the floor, crossing your legs just above your ankles. Observe the height of your knees. If the tops of your knees are higher than your upper pelvic bones, sit on one or two folded blankets. Raising the hips like this allows your pelvis to tilt forward and your spine to be erect without strain.

2. Pull your buttocks, sitting bones, and upper thighs back and apart with your hands. This also enables you to sit up tall with a normal amount of lumbar arch.

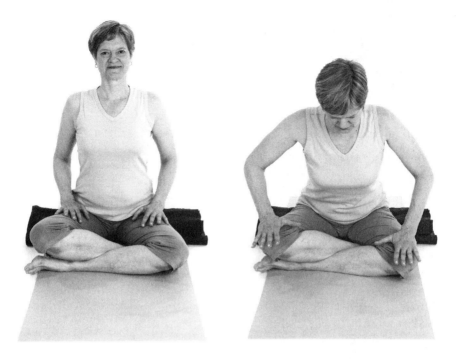

3. Lift up your lower abdomen and root your tailbone down, creating length and support in your lumbar spine.
4. Place your hands on top of your knees.
5. Push up with your legs and down with your hands in an isometric action.
6. Lift up through your torso as you root downward through the pelvic bones.
7. Notice all sensations in your back, hips, and pelvis. You might feel some discomfort at first, which will lessen as the bones realign. Be patient.
8. Change the crossing of your legs (if you had the right one in front of the left, put the left one in front of the right) and then repeat the exercise.

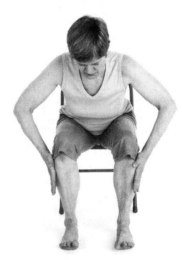

This pose uses isometric strength to widen the pelvic bones.

7. *PRESSURE COOKER—See page 73.

8. *CHAIR TWIST—See page 75.

9. CHAIR GARUDASANA (Eagle Pose)

Purpose: To stretch the iliotibial band and widen the back of the pelvis.

Contraindication: Severe hypertension.

Prop: A chair.

Avoiding pitfalls: If this is painful, stick to Pressure Cooker (page 73) as an alternative.

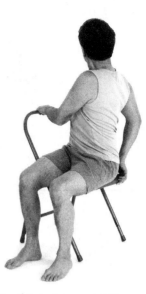

In this twist we stabilize the pelvis while moving the spine, which is a good skill to practice.

INSTRUCTIONS:

1. Sit at the front of a chair and manually widen your buttocks and upper thighs.
2. Cross your right leg over your left, putting the knees in a vertical line.
3. Inhale; lift up your spine.
4. Exhale. Put some strength in your lower abdominal muscles to support your core strength.
5. Isometrically push your thighs apart. This action will firm the sides of your hips and you may feel a stretch in your outer thighs. *Keep breathing!*
6. For more intensity, put your right hand on the outside of your right knee, left hand outside the left knee, and push in with your hands and out with your legs.
7. Release and repeat on the other side.

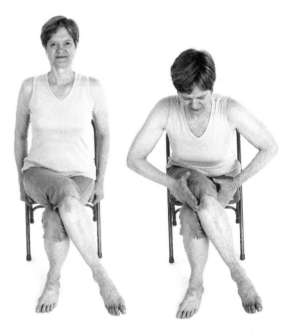

10. *STANDING LUNGE WITH CHAIR—See page 72.

11. STANDING MARICHYASANA III

Purpose: To open the sacroiliac joint, improve strength and mobility of the spine, and refine balance.

Contraindications: Subluxation/dislocation of the hip, total or partial hip replacement.

Props: A yoga mat and a chair.

Avoiding pitfalls: Be mindful of all the alignment details, even if it means that you do not twist as far.

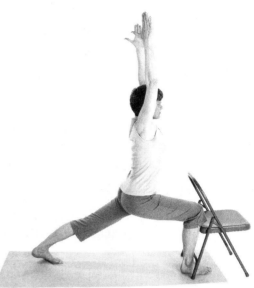

Use the chair to set your alignment and balance. Then complete the pose.

INSTRUCTIONS:

1. Stand facing the seat of a chair, feet parallel and hip-width apart.
2. Place your right foot on the chair seat, with the knee and foot pointing straight forward from the hip.
3. Firm your legs and spinal muscles.
4. Widen your sitting bones apart, tilting the top of the pelvis forward slightly.
5. Move the left top thigh back, and resolve to keep it there as you proceed.
6. Lengthen the tailbone down; add tone and lift your lower abdomen.
7. Place your right hand on your hip and your left hand on your right knee.
8. Inhale, stretch up through your spine, and root down through the left leg.
9. Exhale and turn your spine (above the pelvis) to the right. Pull on your right thigh with your left hand to help the twist. Keep the right thigh firm and wide to resist the pressure of the hand.

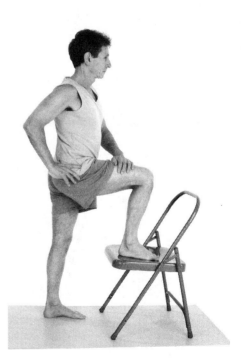

10. Actively wrap your left lower ribs around toward the right, beginning with the back ribs, while keeping your left leg firmly rooted. Resist its tendency to move forward.
11. Keep your shoulders and head level, and intelligently work with moderate effort—not too aggressively, not too gently.
12. Release and repeat on the other side.

12. UTTHITA PARSVAKONASANA (variation with chair)

Purpose: To move the sacroiliac joint, improve hip flexibility, and increase leg and spinal strength while safely supported.

Contraindications: Ischial bursitis, coccygodynia.

Props: A yoga mat and a chair.

Avoiding pitfalls: Adjust for your height relative to the chair if necessary. If your front foot does not easily reach the floor, place a phone book under it. If you are tall, put the phone book on the chair seat. Even though you have a chair for support, work diligently in the pose.

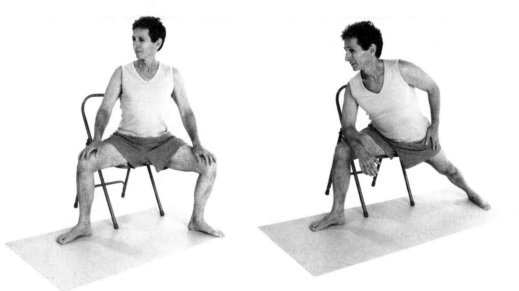

INSTRUCTIONS:

1. Sit on the chair with your legs wide apart.
2. Manually widen your buttocks and upper thighs.
3. Open your right knee out to the side and place your foot directly under the knee.
4. Lean to the right, moving from your hip not your waist, and rest your forearm on your thigh.
5. Move the left leg to the left until it stretches straight, keeping the toes and the knee facing forward. Most of your weight will now be on your right hip.
6. With the muscles of your legs and pelvis active, curl your tailbone diagonally down toward your left foot, along the same angle at which your whole body is now inclined.
7. Firm your abdominal muscles and from the core of your pelvis extend out into both legs and up through your spine.

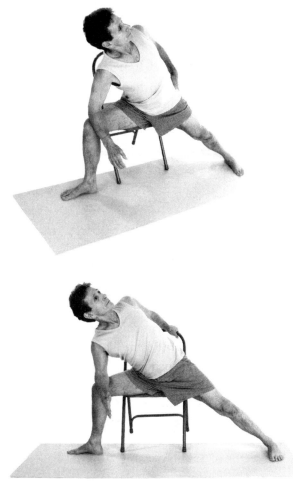

8. Place your left hand on your left hip and roll your left shoulder back until your whole upper body faces forward. Looking up may help you to turn your upper body.
9. For more intensity, turn your torso enough to the left to grasp the back of the chair with your left hand, and look up.
10. Retain the pose for several breaths, and then release and repeat on the other side.

13. LEANING PEACOCK
(Mayurasana variation with table)

Purpose: To use gravity to realign the sacroiliac joints.

Contraindications: Carpal tunnel syndrome, fractured rib, tennis elbow.

Props: A table or desk; an optional yoga mat.

Avoiding pitfalls: Pay attention to the alignment of the rest of the body, especially keeping the shoulders back as much as possible. If your wrists are stiff, use a yoga mat under your hands. Let your lower body really hang. Refrain from using abdominal or lower back muscles.

INSTRUCTIONS:

1. Place your hands on the tabletop, with your palms flat and fingers pointing back toward you and curled under the edge of the table. Your hands should be so close together that your elbows touch the front of the rib cage.

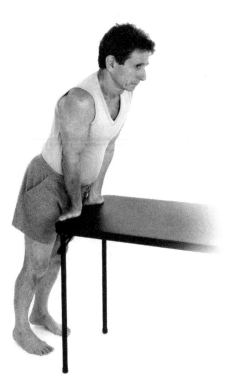

2. Place your feet comfortably apart.
3. Take a deep breath in to lengthen up through your spine.
4. Pull your shoulders back.
5. Keep your arm and upper back muscles firm as you begin to transfer weight to your hands, letting your knees bend. Your elbows should be slightly bent.
6. Totally relax your abdominal and lower back muscles.

7. Allow gravity to pull your pelvis down while you
   hold your chest up.
8. Maintain the pose, breathing normally.
9. Carefully bring your weight back to your legs and
   stand up straight.

14. *ADHO MUKHA SVANASANA (Stage II, Wall Dog)—See page 63.

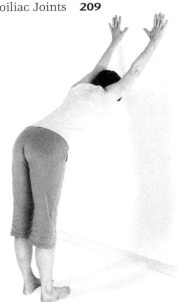

This pose is a good neutralizer after the intense poses just completed.

15. *SETU BANDHASANA—See page 81.

This pose strengthens the back pelvic muscles.

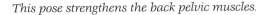

16. GOMUKHASANA LEGS ONLY (with and without resistance from hands)

This pose is similar to Chair Garudasana (page 204), but being on the
floor makes it more intense.

Purpose: To stretch abductors and iliotibial band, to open the
sacroiliac joint.

Contraindications: Absolute: total hip replacement. Relative:
ischial bursitis, total knee replacement.

Props: A mat and one or two folded blankets.

Avoiding pitfalls: Use enough height under your hips to sit up
straight with your pelvis vertical, not sloping back.

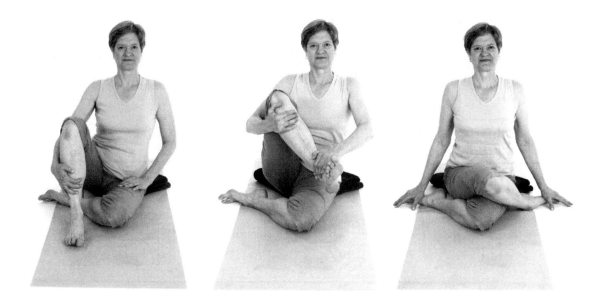

INSTRUCTIONS:

1. Place a folded blanket or two on a mat, with one corner pointing forward.
2. Sit on the front corner of the blanket(s) as shown: left knee pointing forward, right knee up.
3. Grasp your right leg with both hands and cross it over the left.
4. Stack your right knee atop your left, with feet off to the side.
5. If your knees stay very high up, use more support under your hips.
6. Manually move the buttocks apart as much as possible. This will free your pelvis to bend forward.
7. Inhale, lift through your spine, and tone the leg muscles.
8. Isometrically pull your thighs apart without changing their alignment. The resistance of your crossed legs will relax the inner thighs.
9. For more intensity, lean forward, put your right hand just above your right knee, and your left hand just above your left knee.

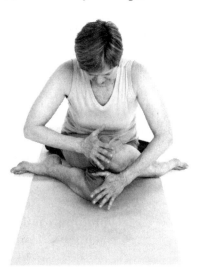

10. Push in with your hands and out with your thighs—a stronger iso-metric action.
11. Breathe smoothly during this intense action.
12. Release, unfold your legs, and change sides.

---

17. *JANU SIRSASANA (with belt)— See page 91.

---

18. MARICHYASANA I (Seated Forward Bend with Push-Pull Action)

Purpose: To use the leverage of the arms and legs to align the sacroiliac joint.

Contraindications: Vertebral fracture, extreme stiffness.

Props: One or two folded blankets to sit on, and a belt.

Avoiding pitfalls: Do not force this one. Use your strength, but use it gradually and symmetrically. Be sure to adjust the pelvis manually as per instruction 2.

INSTRUCTIONS:

1. Sit on the edge of the folded blanket(s) with your legs extended forward, hip-width apart. Have your belt handy.
2. Manually widen your but-tocks and hamstring mus-cles, while keeping the leg position. This will greatly help you to tip the pelvis forward, which is crucial in this pose.
3. Bend your left knee up, your shin nearly vertical, and place your left foot in close to your left hip.

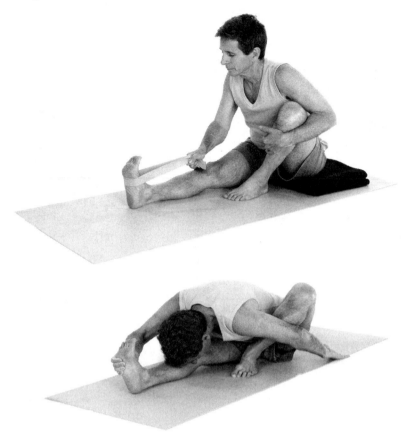

4. Pause and breathe, lifting up with strength in your back.
5. Root your right thigh down toward the floor, and press the heel forward without actually moving it.
6. Inhale and lengthen up again through your back.
7. Exhaling, bend forward. If you can, place your left upper arm in front of your left shin. Otherwise, grasp your left shin with your left hand.
8. With your right hand, reach for your right foot; use a belt if you need to.
9. Create a push-pull action: pull on your outstretched foot or the belt with your right hand, and push on your left shin with your left arm. Both actions move the torso forward.
10. For more intensity, bring your head down to your leg and wrap your left upper arm around the front of the left shin. Wrap the left hand and forearm back behind you. This will strengthen the push-pull action.
11. Maintain this action for several breaths, then release and change sides.

19. *JATHARA PARIVARTANASANA—See page 84.

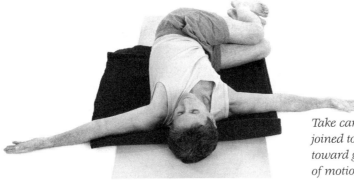

Take care to keep the legs actively joined together. Progress carefully toward greater side-to-side range of motion.

20. PIGEON POSE (Eka Pada Rajakapotasana, preparation with chair and bolster)

Purpose: To improve sacroiliac nutation and hip flexibility, specifically the iliotibial band, gluteal muscles, quadriceps, and iliopsoas (hip extensors and flexors).

Contraindications: Spondylolisthesis, spinal stenosis, vertebral fracture, iliopsoas bursitis, total hip replacement.

Props: A yoga mat, blanket, chair, and bolster. Eliminate the bolster if your flexibility allows.

Avoiding pitfalls: Add a folded blanket on top of the bolster if you need more height.

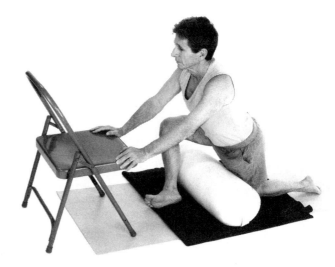

INSTRUCTIONS:

1. Facing the chair, lower yourself onto a bolster. Your right leg goes in front of it and your left leg behind. Your left knee will be on the floor.

2. Move your right knee to

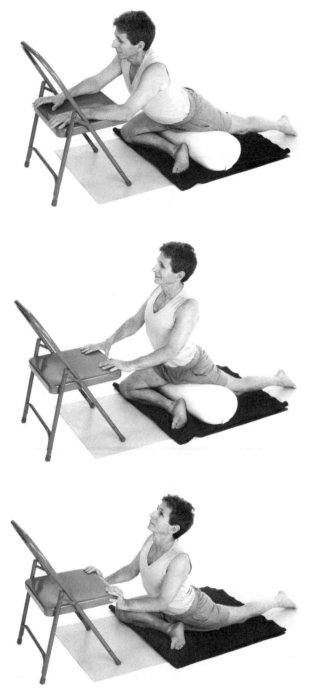

the side about forty-five degrees; line up your right foot in front of your left hip.

3. Lean on the chair with your arms to be able to adjust your pelvis and legs more easily.

4. Stretch your left leg back, turning it to face your knee downward and your pelvis straight forward toward the chair. Orient your toes straight back.

5. To square your hips, pull the left one forward and the right one back.

6. Inhale, lift up through your torso, and firm the muscles of your legs.

7. Reach your sitting bones and upper thighs back and apart, which will temporarily arch your lower back.

8. Exhale, lower yourself fully onto the bolster, and curl your tailbone down to lengthen the lower back.

9. From the core of your pelvis, stretch up strongly through your spine and root down through the pelvic bones and legs.

10. For more stretch in the back leg, remove the bolster and lift your torso higher.

11. For more stretch in the front leg, lean forward toward the chair.

12. In either case, keep your pelvis square to the front.

13. While holding the pose, breathe and fully stretch through your

spine and legs, even into your feet. Most people feel the most intense stretch in the buttock of the front leg.

14. To exit the pose, roll toward the right and bring your left leg forward.
15. Repeat on the other side.

21. *CHILD'S POSE—See page 92.

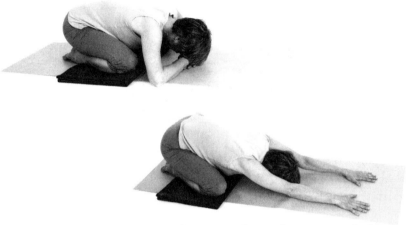

Rest in this pose with your legs symmetrical.

22. *SAVASANA

Follow the instructions on pages 93–94, with this addition: put a belt loosely around your legs, either just above or just below the knees, to keep the legs more parallel. This will protect the sacroiliac joints.

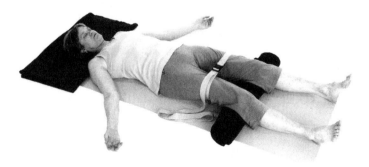

Sacroiliac *Asana*: Types of Motion and Function

Name	Nutation	ROM Vertical	ROM Lateral	ROM Anterior-Posterior	Stability	Torque
Tadasana with Block		1	2			
*Windshield Wiper	3	1	1			1
*Lotus Prep with Wall			1		1	1
*Supta Padangusthasana	2[a]	2			2	1
Bhujangasana	1	1	1	1	1	
Sukhasana	1	1	3		1	
*Pressure Cooker	1	3	3	1	1	
*Chair Twist	2		1		1	2
Chair Garudasana			3	1		
*Standing Lunge with Chair	2[a]	3			1	1
Standing Marichyasana III	2[a]	1	1		1	1
Utthita Parsvakonasana	3	1	1			2
Leaning Peacock		2				
*Wall Dog		3	1	2		
*Setu Bandhasana		1		2	2	
Gomukhasana Legs Only	1[a]	1	3	1		
*Janu Sirsasana	2[a]	1	1	1		1
Marichyasana I	2[a]	1	1	1		1
*Jathara Parivartanasana	2		1			2
Pigeon Pose	2[a]	1	1			1
*Child's Pose		1		1		
*Savasana	None					

Note: Nutation is nodding, a back-and-forth motion. We define this to include diagonal motion in the sacroiliac joint: if the left superior corner of the sacrum goes forward, then the right inferior portion goes back. ROM = range of motion. Numbers indicate degree of intensity: 1 = moderate; 2 = substantial; 3 = near maximal.

[a]Nutation due to assymetry of pose.

CHAPTER 12

The Wrists and Hands

Our hands are possibly more characteristic of our humanity than are our faces. We need them to hold cell phones and ice cream cones, to button and unbutton, to make beds and play billiards, to type on keyboards, to give change, to make food and almost anything else. The structure of our hands has very likely evolved to meet our survival needs. And marvelously complex and well integrated they are, with tendons attached to tendons across dozens of small bones and joints. Parts of the brain have developed apace, with motor cells in the cortex executing movements, and sensory cells just behind them monitoring what the hands have gotten themselves into. It is a fine example of evolution, or rather co-evolution: controller (the brain) and executor (the hands) each enabling the other's further refinement.

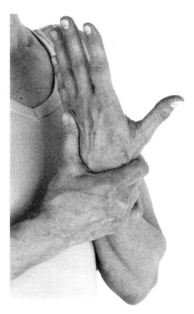

Because of their ubiquitous utility, the hands, too, are prime prey of a disease based on wear and tear. Yoga is useful in its characteristic ways: improving range of motion, enhancing the health of the many joints, providing stretch and calm to inflamed parts.

Because of the hands' many joints and multijoint interactions (think of the opposition of the thumb), yoga provides fertile ground on which to practice stretching of the ligaments, tendons, capsules, and muscles. The only caveat is not to go too far too fast. The muscles and joints of the wrist and hand are no match for their larger and more powerful neighbors situated closer to the shoulder. Caution and sensitivity are the keys to successful work here.

It is easy to improve the dexterity and sensitivity of painless and more capable joints, but the best part of dexterity improvement comes from unmitigated concentration on the details of exercises like those that follow. You may have to move through stiffness and discomfort. Trust yourself to distinguish between the unpleasant but healthful action of moving stiff joints, and the discomfort of straining a structure beyond its capacity.

Coordination of seemingly disparate tasks is the soul of dexterity. In the hand it is a three-dimensional matter. Consider holding a paint brush: two fingers bend and rise, one pulls inward and curves while the thumb applies a gentle downward pressure and the wrist turns inward—this all to simply hold the brush, never mind actually painting. Compare this with the spine, where the long row of vertebrae share three planes of movement, but always in a linear relationship.

Because the hands are connected to the arms and ultimately the trunk, all shoulder poses and neck poses can help with hand and wrist problems. Especially remember the Shoulder Loop (see page 99), which gives essential support to the arms in all poses. Also think of the hand having four corners just as the foot does—especially when the hand is on a surface such as the floor or a wall, but also in poses like Parsvottanasana Prep (arms only), described below. In some poses it may help to imagine the contact with one or more of the corners.

Most muscles that move the wrist, hand, and fingers are not located there, but in the forearm. Finer movements and adjustments would be greatly obstructed by the bulk of the muscles were they located in the hand itself, and by the momentum that such weight in the hand would generate. Therefore, the tendons that move the fingers pull over many joints to reach the muscles that control them. Have you ever seen an aerial view of a train accident? The cars are aligned in zigzag fashion. Forces a little off center on one car move it to the right. This forces the next car to the left, and the one after that to the right. The same thing happens in severe arthritis of the hand. The only difference is that in arthritis of the hand, the asymmetry of forces seems to originate from changes in the joints themselves (even though the forces come from far away in the forearm).

Fortunately, the soft tissue elements in the hand hold things together. The *intrinsic muscles* of the hand, those actually beginning and ending in the hand, are often attached to the tendons of the longer muscles that originate in the forearm, and mitigate their potentially overpowering pull. Also, the *fibrocartilaginous triangle* and other, less dramatically conservative structures restrain the hand's malformation.

Our goal is to keep the hand in good form by increasing its ranges of motion at the different joints. The idea is that if the forces to one side and the other can be relatively equalized, contrary to the uneven deviations promoted by arthritis (remember the image of the train wreck), then symmetry can be maintained. In addition, greater range of motion will, of course, directly counter the losses of dexterity that come along with arthritis.

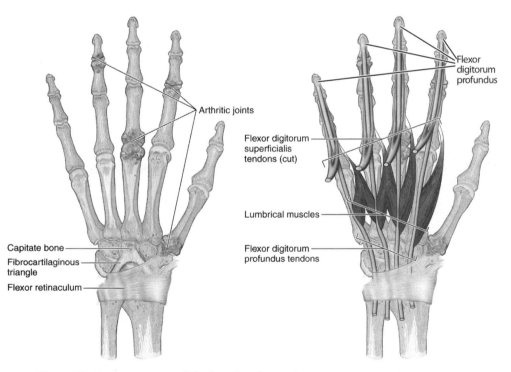

Figure 11. *Basic structure of the hand: palmar views.*

Poses

1. DIGITAL ROLY POLY

Purpose: To coordinate and mobilize all the finger and wrist joints with multidirectional movement.

Contraindications: Active gout, pseudogout, volar or intertriginous dermatitis.

Props: None.

Avoiding pitfalls: Start slowly, stay loose!

INSTRUCTIONS:

1. Sitting or standing, hold your hands at a comfortable height in front of you. Interlace your fingers.
2. Make fluid figure-of-eight shapes with your wrists, moving at a comfortable speed and with as little tension as possible in your fingers.
3. Do ten repetitions.
4. Reverse the direction of the figure-of-eight and repeat.

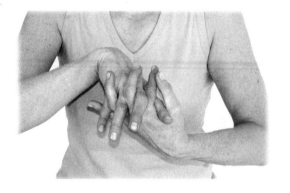 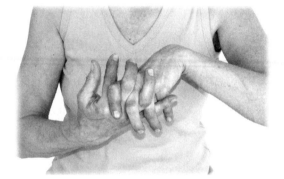

2. FINGER PUSH-UPS

Purpose: To strengthen the muscles that flex the fingers, and increase range of motion for flexion.

Contraindication: Dupuytren's contracture.

Props: A table and chair or a wall.

Avoiding pitfalls: Keep your shoulders pulled back, and position yourself relative to the table to allow your upper arms to hang by your sides without strain.

INSTRUCTIONS:

1. Place your hands flat on a table or wall. Sit up tall with your shoulders back and wide.
2. Push your fingers into the table or wall, so that your wrists lift off. Keeping your fingers slightly curved, raise your wrists as far as you can, gathering all five fingers in toward each other.
3. Flatten your hand again to repeat the action five to ten times.

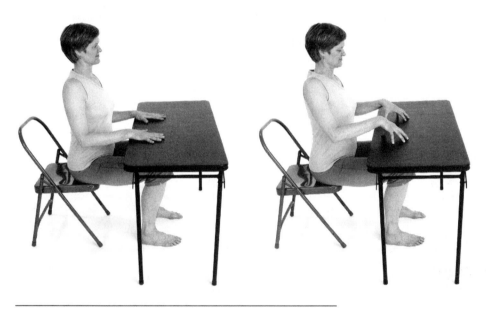

3. ANJALI MUDRA SERIES (Prayer Position)

Purpose: To improve wrist extension at varying angles, which will stretch the wrist flexor muscles, and increase mobility of the carpal and metacarpal bones.

Contraindication: Dupuytren's contracture.

Prop: Possibly a chair; this pose can be done sitting or standing.

Avoiding pitfalls: Retract your shoulders; keep the front of your chest open.

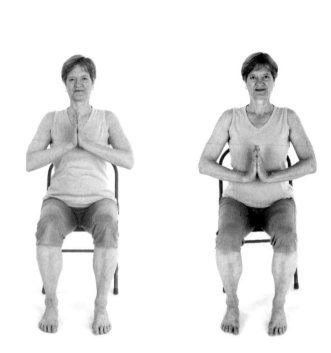

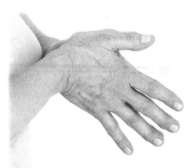

INSTRUCTIONS:

1. Sitting or standing, join your palms together as high up in the air as you can, perhaps just overhead. Press the four corners of the palms together.

2. Retain the strong connection of the palms and slowly lower them until they are in front of your chest. Pause there, with your fingers angled away from your body at a forty-five-degree angle.

3. Turn your fingertips up and in toward your body, pointing the fingers straight up.

4. Gently push your wrists down as far as possible without separating the heels of the hands.

5. Stay in this position for fifteen seconds, retaining the retracted shoulders.

6. Turn your hands and fingertips away from your body and down, wrists staying in close to you.

7. Press your palms together in this position for fifteen seconds, then release.

4. UNSEEN STAFF (Wrist Flexion)

Purpose: To stretch the wrist extensor muscles.

Contraindications: de Quervain's syndrome, tennis elbow.

Props: None.

Avoiding pitfalls: Keep your shoulders pulled back and your overall posture tall and open.

INSTRUCTIONS:

1. Extend your right hand straight out in front of you, palm facing in.
2. Curl your fingers into a loose fist, as if holding a staff.
3. Use your left hand to curl the right fingers and hand in toward the inner arm, until you feel a good stretch on the outside of your right wrist.
4. Keep your elbow straight and the inner elbow crease turned toward the left, not up.
5. Hold with patience and care for about thirty seconds.
6. Release and repeat on the other side.

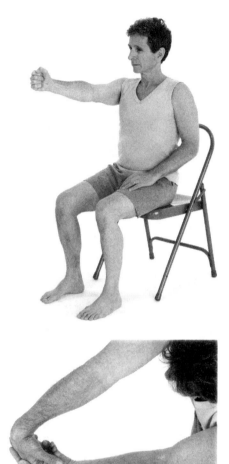

5. EKA DIGITAL FLEXION
(flexing each joint of one finger at a time)

Purpose: To improve range of motion of each finger's flexion.

Contraindication: Golfer's elbow.

Props: A chair and table.

Avoiding pitfalls: Do not be too forceful; mild resistance will be enough to reap the benefits of this pose.

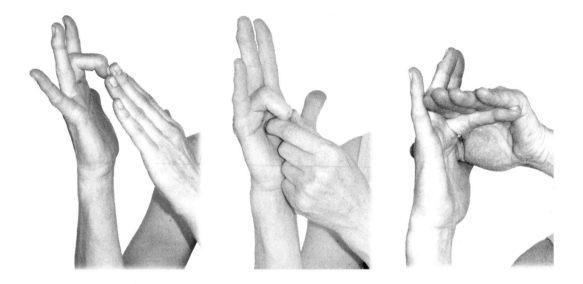

INSTRUCTIONS:

1. Sit comfortably, possibly with your elbows on a desk or table, palms facing you.

2. One finger at a time, bend each joint in toward the palm. First bend the distal joint, then the middle one, and then the proximal one, each time giving pressure with your other hand. Steady the palm so that the action is specific in the finger joints.

3. Work through each finger of each hand thoroughly, then open and close your fists a few times.

---

6. STOP (distant relative of Vasisthasana)

Purpose: To stretch the wrist and finger flexors, biceps, brachialis, latissimus dorsi, teres major, and pectoral muscles.

Contraindications: Fibrocartilaginous triangle injury (sprain or more serious), voluntary shoulder subluxation, severe wrist arthritis.

Prop: A wall.

Avoiding pitfalls: Place your hand directly to your side on the wall, not behind you. Keep your muscles firm but not rigid, and your elbow slightly bent, not locked straight.

INSTRUCTIONS:

1. Stand with your left side about eighteen inches away from a wall.
2. Place your left hand on the wall, with your index finger pointing upward and palm flat, directly to your side and not behind you. Press the four corners of your palm into the wall.
3. Take a breath to expand inside your chest. Stand tall.
4. Gently retract your right shoulder, sliding the shoulder blade in toward the spine.
5. Use a moderate amount of strength to press into the wall.
6. Turn your feet in place to face your body away from the wall.
7. Stop turning when you feel a good stretch in the palm and/or across your upper chest and shoulder. For more stretch, straighten your elbow.
8. Hold for a few breaths.
9. Remove your hand from the wall, keeping its shape, and hold this for five seconds.
10. Repeat on the right side.

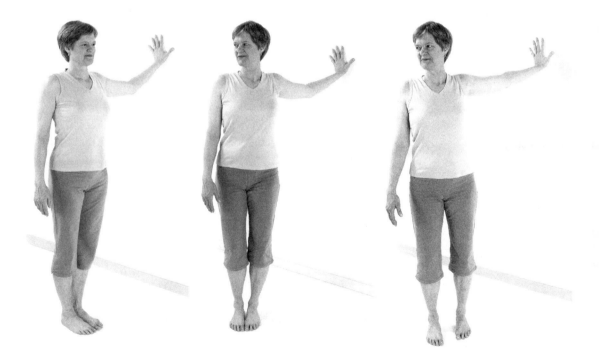

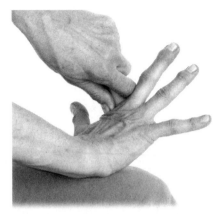

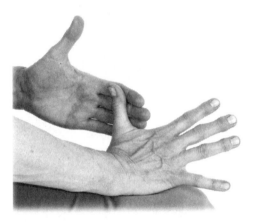

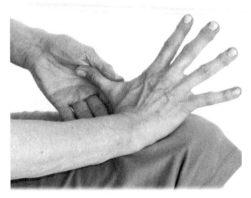

7. EKA DIGITAL EXTENSION

Purpose: To maintain the ability to stretch the fingers straight.

Contraindication: Dupuytren's contracture.

Prop: A chair.

Avoiding pitfalls: Pull your shoulders back and sit tall to avoid excess tension in the neck and shoulders.

INSTRUCTIONS:

1. While sitting, put your right hand on your right thigh, with your fingers pointing inward toward the left.
2. Hold your right index finger with the left hand. Place your left thumb at the knuckle of your right index finger.
3. Use the thumb as a fulcrum to raise the finger up and stretch the finger back. Gently press down at the knuckle and the wrist.
4. Stretch each finger. Hold the full range of motion for at least ten seconds.
5. Pull the thumb up twice, once closer to the index finger, once out perpendicular to it and the wrist.
6. Repeat on the left side.

8. AIKIDO WRIST STRETCHES

We suggest two variations of this pose.

Supinate and Twist

Purpose: To stretch the wrist, hand, and forearm with flexion and supination combined.

Contraindications: de Quervain's syndrome, severe osteoporosis, pseudogout.

Props: None.

Avoiding pitfalls: Maintain good Tadasana posture with your whole body: shoulders back, chest broad, spine long.

INSTRUCTIONS:

1. Place your left hand near the center of your chest. Turn the palm toward the left, thumb pointing out away from you.
2. Grasp the base of the left wrist with your right hand; place your right thumb at the back of the hand near the base of the left little finger.
3. Pull your wrist down along your midline. Keep it facing sideways, finger still pointing up, until the forearm is horizontal.
4. Repeat several times, moving up and down to explore the range of movement. Be curious but do not look for trouble. Breathe smoothly and remember the Shoulder Loop (see page 99).
5. Repeat with the other arm.

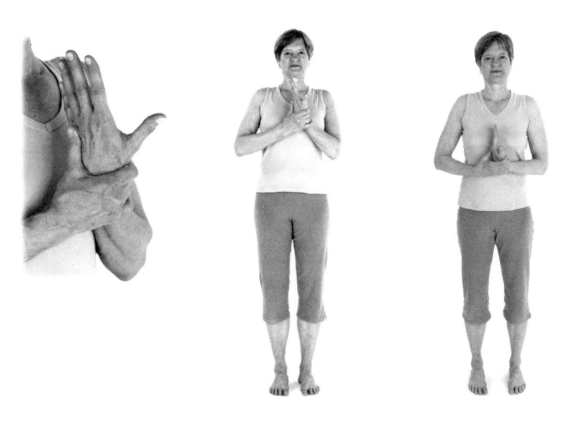

Pronate and Twist

Purpose: To stretch the wrist and forearm, combining flexion with pronation.

Contraindications: Severe osteoporosis, pseudogout.

Props: None.

Avoiding pitfalls: Maintain good Tadasana posture with your whole body: shoulders back, chest broad, spine long.

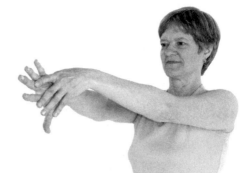

INSTRUCTIONS:

1. Raise your right arm before you, with your thumb pointing down.
2. Position your left hand over the top of the right hand, with your thumb on the palm and your fingers on the back of the hand.
3. Use your left hand to stabilize the right and retain this orientation as you bend your right elbow to the side, pulling the right wrist in toward you.
4. Go over this in-and-out movement several times at a comfortable speed. Gently expand the range of motion in your wrist and forearm.
5. Repeat, with the hands reversed.

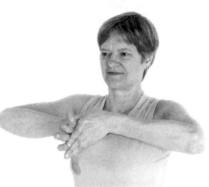

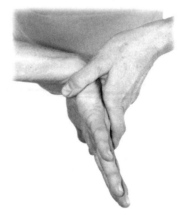

9. WALL FINGER STRETCH

Purpose: To stretch the palm and extend all eight fingers together.

Contraindications: Dupuytren's contracture, damage to the fibrocartilaginous triangle.

Prop: A wall.

Avoiding pitfalls: Remember the shoulder principles—Inner Body Bright, Muscular Energy, Shoulder Loop, and Organic Energy (see page 99).

INSTRUCTIONS:

1. Place your fingertips on the wall at about eye level.
2. Lift up from inside, firm your arm muscles, and pull your shoulder blades toward the spine.
3. Slowly push your fingers flat onto the wall, but pull back with your palms.
4. Balance the pushing in with the pulling back.
5. For more intensity, start with your hands lower on the wall.
6. Hold the stretch for thirty seconds, then release.

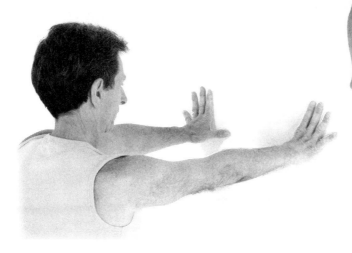

10. PARSVOTTANASANA PREP (Arms Only)

Purpose: To stretch the wrists, fingers, and forearms.

Contraindications: Subluxation of the radial head, Dupuytren's contracture.

Props: None.

Avoiding pitfalls: Maintain good Tadasana posture with your whole body. Retract the shoulders slightly.

INSTRUCTIONS:

1. Stand tall and bring your hands to your waist, with your shoulders back and chest broad.
2. Catch your fingertips, facing upward, on the back of your pelvis near your waistline.
3. As you inhale, expand upward through your torso.
4. Exhale. Push your wrists down as far as possible. Aim to keep the fingers pointing straight up. Point your elbows straight back.
5. Hold for ten to fifteen seconds, then gently release.

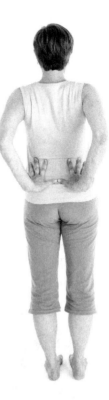

---

11. *TADASANA URDHVA BADDHA HASTASANA—See page 60.

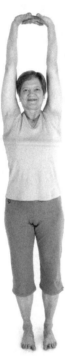

This pose provides a full stretch of the shoulders, arms, and hands.

Wrist and Hand *Asana*: Types of Motion and Intensity

Name	Finger					Wrist					
	Flexion	Extension	Abduction	Adduction	Neutral	Flexion	Extension	Radial Deviation	Ulnar Deviation	Pronation	Supination
Digital Roly Poly	1	1	1	1		1	1	1	1	1	1
Finger Push-ups	2	1		1	2	2				1	
Anjali Mudra Series		2	1				2	1	1	2	2
Unseen Staff	3			1		3	1				
Eka Digital Flexion	3				2						
Stop		2	2		2		3			1	
Eka Digital Extension		2	2								
Aikido Wrist Stretch: Supinate and Twist		2			2	2			2[a]		3
Aikido Wrist Stretch: Pronate and Twist			1		1	3			3	3	
Wall Finger Stretch		2									
Parsvottanasana Prep		3					3	1		2	
*Tadasana Urdhva Baddha Hastasana		3	1				3			3	

[a] Can be done in neutral.

CHAPTER 13

The Feet and Ankles

The feet and ankles have a peculiar relationship with us humans. Possibly because we walk upright, the hands, with their almost uniquely human abilities to write, make complex gestures, and use tools, have an elevated status all their own, whereas the "lower" parts of our anatomy are regarded with the opposite sentiment. However, human feet are anatomically interesting in their own right, and exactly because we are bipeds, they undergo stresses and suffer consequent damages that are uniquely their own.

Typically, men correct their balance by adjusting their hips, while women maintain their stability with their ankles.[1] It is not clear whether this is due to the reluctance of girls of previous generations to engage in hip-intensive athletics; to feminine shoes that have higher heels and therefore require ankle agility; or to other factors. Again, with maintaining balance, the principles of cooperation apply; the

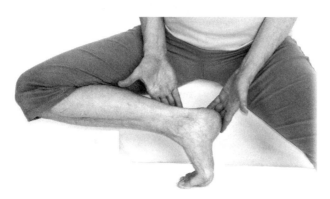

hips have very wide ranges of motion yet little capacity to take the shock of abrupt compression, while the one-dimensional movement of the knees provides resilience and shock absorption by virtue of the great strength of the muscles that cross them. These two joints, and the torso as a whole, can compensate for increased stress on the feet by easing momentary impacts, reducing disadvantageous angling, and redistributing weight during routine, repetitive tasks such as walking, negotiating stairs, and stopping abruptly.

Walking is a very complex activity in which the feet themselves, as well as their many parts, do a lot of adapting. In normal walking, the ankle flexes and extends twice for every step, transferring all the weight onto each foot with the forward movement of the other, and requiring medial-lateral stability throughout the gait cycle. Descending stairs,

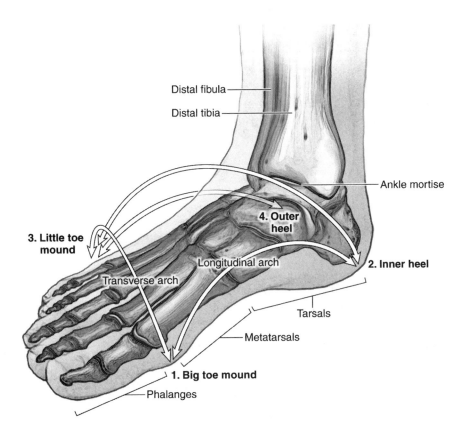

Figure 12. *Arches of the foot.*

walking with a stone in the left shoe, stepping on a roof, breaking in new shoes—all oblige us to adapt and alter this normal motion.

With every step we take, the distribution of weight on our feet varies instantaneously. Dr. Renee Cailliet divides the foot into twelve parts: if one were allotting twelve pounds of weight while standing on one foot, it would be six for the heel, two for the big toe, and one for each of the other toes along with the corresponding parts of the ball of the foot.[2] But this only holds for standing still. The changes that occur in quite normal walking are more complex.

There are twenty-seven bones and thirty-two joints in each foot, and osteoarthritis commonly befalls them. Arthritic difficulties in the foot range from a bunion to degenerative joint disease, with its characteristic limitations of range of motion, swelling, and pain; to the joint disorders that come from the chronic "abuse" of women's footwear and obesity; to the most acute and extreme joint disruptions that originate in fracture and sprain.

In these pages we address limitations in range of motion and instability, which derive from muscle and tendon shortening and muscular weakness. Our purpose is to enliven your awareness and your abilities to adapt. We work on each motion of the foot's many parts, but you must bear in mind that range of motion, strength, and coordination of the knees, hips, and lower back are relevant to the happiness of the feet. For that reason you will see some hip-opening poses in this chapter.

Mr. Iyengar often directs students' attention to the feet and toes. His beautiful and powerful standing poses are, of course, based on support, balance, and exact mastery of the feet. The instructions in this chapter embody many of his methods. The emphasis by Anusara Yoga on weight distribution is an excellent place to start. When you are standing, Anusara Yoga recommends balancing your weight at the four corners of the feet, which will ensure that the intrinsic muscles of the feet are active. First, root the big toe mound, then the inner heel, then the little toe mound, then the outer heel. You will probably find yourself less aware of one or more of these corners than the others, but with practice you will find a balance between them. From this steady foundation, the rest of the body (and your disposition) can have the support for all that yoga requires.

Stability of each foot also depends on the knee and the tibia. Moving the base of the shin bone backward while lifting the arch further stabilizes the ankle. One quick and easy way to begin to establish these actions in the feet is to lift up all ten toes, while the balls of the feet stay down. When you are doing this, the arches will naturally lift, the heels will press down, and the base of the shin bone will move back, an action that is part of the Ankle Loop (see Appendix III). Again press the balls of the feet down, which will tone the back of the lower leg. This is the Shin Loop (see Appendix III). The action of a large lower leg muscle, the gastrocnemius, will help to prevent hyperextension of the knee.

There are two common pitfalls that apply to all the poses for the feet and ankles, and so we list them here, with their remedies.

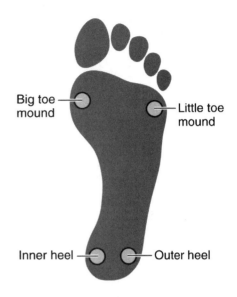

Figure 13. *The foot's four points of support. When standing, weight should be evenly distributed among these four points.*

- Collapsed inner arch: The remedy is to lift your toes and bring more weight to the outer heel.
- Sickled foot (the little toe side of the foot curls toward the midline, overstretching the outer ankle): The remedy is to pull the fourth and fifth toes back toward your outer ankles, and align the center of the ankle with the second toe.

---

1. *TADASANA (with special attention to the four corners of the feet)— See page 59.

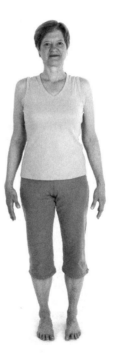

2. *STANDING LUNGE WITH WALL—See page 60.

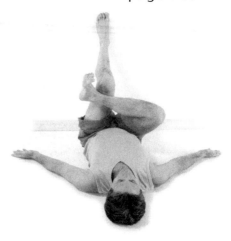

3. *SUPTA PADANGUSTHASANA—See page 83.

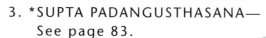

Ankle and toe flexors that do not cross the knee are stretched in the forward leg; ankle flexors that cross the knee are stretched in the back leg.

4. *LOTUS PREP WITH WALL—See page 78.

Stretching the entire leg in this pose helps coordinate the actions of the hip, knee, and foot while standing and walking.

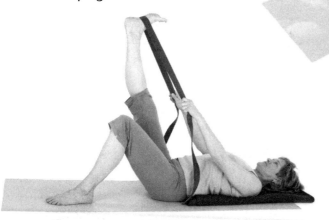

Tight hamstring muscles strain the lower back.

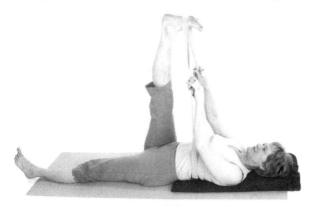

Better movement range in the deep hip muscles enables us to balance better on the feet.

5. UTKATASANA

Purpose: To align and strengthen the quadriceps, adductors, and abductors and to coordinate ankles, knees, hips, and lumbar spine in common balancing movements. To extend the ankles.

Contraindications: Imbalance, acromioclavicular subluxation, rotator cuff tear, severe osteoporosis, profound weakness, anterior cruciate tear, advanced chondromalacia patellae.

Prop: A wall.

Avoiding pitfalls: Take care to align the knees so the kneecaps track straight forward over the second toes, and to align the lower back without either arching or curving it excessively.

INSTRUCTIONS:

1. Stand a few feet from a wall, facing it.
2. Reach your arms forward, shoulder-width apart. Place your fingertips lightly on the wall above eye level.
3. Pull your arms deeply into the shoulder sockets. Stretch your legs and draw your abdomen in toward your core with determination.
4. Lift your toes and root your heels down. Balance your weight on the four corners of your feet (see page 235).
5. While inhaling, raise your upper body up from the inside, arching your lower back slightly.
6. Exhale, bend your knees, and reach your hips back. Make one long line from fingers to hips.
7. Widen your thighs apart, as in Pressure Cooker (page 73), without widening the lower legs. Your arms will lean more firmly on the wall.
8. Curl your tailbone down and lift your lower abdomen. This will support your lower back

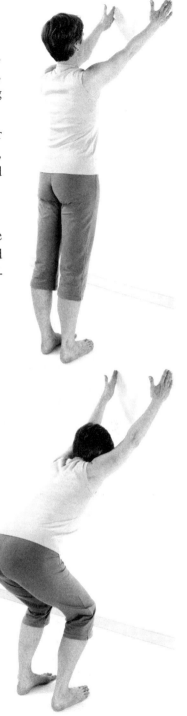

and lessen the arch there. Take special care that the knees track straight forward.

9. Splay the toes apart.
10. Breathe strongly to energize the pose.
11. Inhale as your return to standing.

This pose brings inner and outer strength.

---

6. UTTANASANA WITH ROLLED BLANKET

Purpose: To stretch the ankles, feet, and calves in dorsiflexion.

Contraindications: Herniated lumbar disc, severe imbalance.

Props: A rolled blanket and possibly two blocks.

Avoiding pitfalls: Test out different heights of the roll and choose the one that is best for you.

INSTRUCTIONS:

1. Roll up a blanket. Place the balls of your feet on the blanket, hip-width apart and parallel. Distribute your weight equally on the four corners of each foot.
2. Bend your knees and make sure your heels touch the floor. You can adjust the size of the roll accordingly.

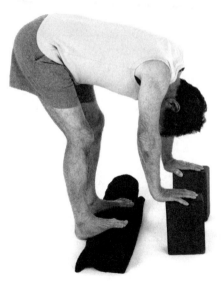

3. Bring your upper body forward as much as possible, with your knees still bent. Touch the floor or two blocks.

4. Take a full easy breath to prepare.

5. Move your shins toward each other and widen your thighs apart.

6. Straighten your knees as much as possible. Adjust your upper body forward enough to bring your hips more over your ankles.

7. Widen your sitting bones as you stretch your legs straighter and straighter. Pull in your abdomen.

8. Root down through the legs all the way into your heels and into the floor as you continue to stretch the sitting bones up.

9. Breathe into the stretch. Be steadfast and patient.

10. To come out of the pose, step off the roll, bend your knees, bring your hands to your hips, and inhale as you come up.

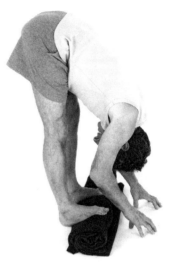

Note: The next four poses stretch and strengthen the hips and legs. Improving their coordination diminishes stress on the ankles and feet.

---

7. *UTTHITA PARSVAKONASANA—See page 67.

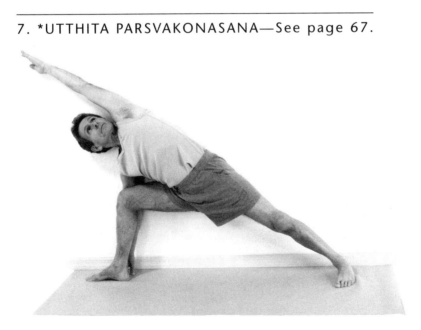

8. *UTTHITA TRIKONASANA— See page 69.

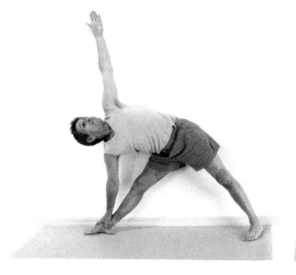

9. *PRASARITA PADOTTANASANA— See page 71.

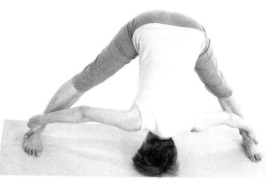

10. *ADHO MUKHA SVANASANA— See page 62.

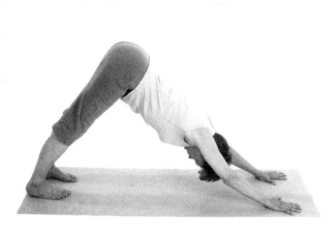

11. *WALL QUAD—See page 76.

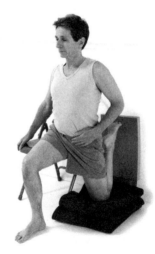

This strong thigh stretch also addresses tightness across the front of the ankle and prepares you for the next pose.

12. VIRASANA (Hero Pose)

Purpose: To stretch the front of the ankles, improve the transverse arch and avoid metatarsalgia.

Contraindications: Total hip replacement, medial or lateral meniscal tear, chondromalacia patellae, medial collateral ligamentous sprain, anterior or posterior cruciate ligamentous sprain, ankle sprain.

Props: A yoga mat, a block, a blanket or two, two washcloths.

Avoiding pitfalls: Experiment to get the right combination of support to stretch your ankles and knees. Avoid sharp pain.

INSTRUCTIONS:

1. Roll a blanket, fold two washcloths, and place all props as shown.

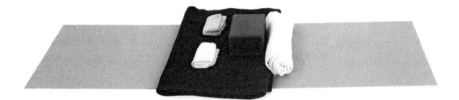

2. Sit on the block with your feet folded back next to your hips. If your ankles are stiff, place them over the rolled blanket. If it is uncomfortable for your knees, add height to the block by placing a folded blanket under it, or use two blocks. Be cautious: there is no need to rush into doing this pose in its classical form.

3. Come up onto your knees and manually pull your calf muscles from the top near the knee down toward your ankles,

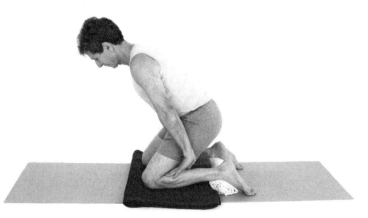

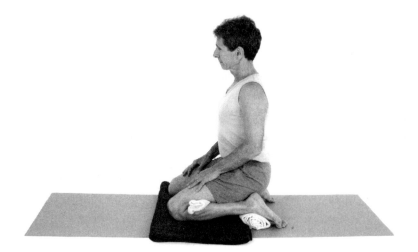

spreading them evenly. Move the muscles (but not the bones) out-ward if painless; use washcloths if needed. This lets the knees fold more easily.

4. Align your feet straight back, in line with your shins. Spread your toes, especially the fourth and fifth toes, and avoid sickling the feet. Sit upright and press the ankles in toward the hips and spread the toes back and apart.

5. Widen your sitting bones and sit tall.

6. Root down through the pelvis and simultaneously rise up through your spine, embodying the dignity of the hero that this pose is named for.

13. MULABANDHASANA
(two stages—one foot or both feet)

Purpose: To stretch toes and ankles, separately and together.

Contraindications: Sacroiliac derangement, knee instability, pes anserinus bursitis, sprained ankle.

Prop: A chair or low stool, possibly a block.

Avoiding pitfalls: Work carefully. Use your hands to guide the position of the foot.

INSTRUCTIONS:

Stage I: One Foot

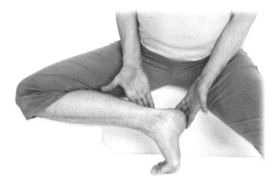

1. Sit in a chair or on a stool or large cushion, with your right knee and foot out to the side.
2. Bend your right knee and place the right foot on the floor at your midline, sole facing to the left, toes bent to the right. With your toes on the floor, lift the ankle and heel up so they come vertically over the big toe. This will create a strong stretch from the Achilles tendon to the tips of your toes.
3. Adjust your posture to root the pelvic bones down and lift the spine.
4. Push your heel away from you with your hands. Aim the knee out to the side and the sole of your foot in toward the midline. This stretches the muscles and connective tissue in the foot and ankle still further, as well as the toe muscles that are intrinsic to the foot.
5. To intensify: Sit lower toward the floor, on a block, and bring the foot close in toward your pelvis with the knee farther to the side.

Stage II: Both Feet

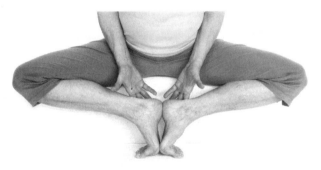

1. Sitting on a block or cushion, bring the soles of the feet together as much as possible, with the toes curled under and pointing out to each side.
2. Press the soles of the feet toward each other, and manually lift the ankles and heels up, stretching the toes. Move the heels away from you so they stack over the big toes.
3. Be patient and careful; use discretion about how much stretch your feet can tolerate.
4. Remember to breathe.

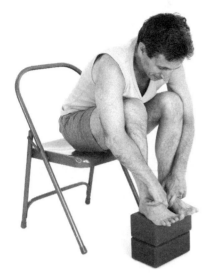

14. TOE ABDUCTION

Purpose: To strengthen the muscles that will reduce and/or prevent bunions.

Contraindications: None.

Props: A chair and two blocks if they make it easier to reach your feet.

Avoiding pitfalls: Intense concentration will help you activate the muscles that move the toes as instructed. Be patient if it is not easy at first. Avoid moving your feet and knees as you isolate this action.

INSTRUCTIONS:

1. Sit in a chair, feet together. Your feet can be on the floor or elevated on blocks for easier access.
2. Lean forward and touch the inner arches of your feet with your fingers. This is the location of the abductor hallucis muscle, which will help the big toe to track straight forward.
3. Now reposition your hands as in the photo, with your index fingers on the inner edges of your big toes, and your thumbs on the inner arches.
4. Push your toes inward against your fingers. Resist the action with your fingers.

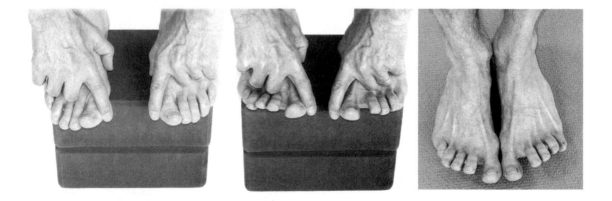

5. With your thumbs feel for the contracting muscle along the inner arches. It is at the back of the arch, in line with the inner ankle bone. Repeat the action five to ten times at first, but practice until you are doing it twenty-five to fifty times. Do it daily.

6. After a few weeks of practice, try this pose while standing up instead of sitting. Stand with the balls of your feet touching, big toes apart. Move the big toes together. It is fine if the toes lift up as you move them, but do not move your feet as a whole or your ankles or knees. The most helpful way to avoid bunions is to incorporate this action into walking.

15. LEGS UP THE WALL

Purpose: To rest the legs and improve foot circulation by providing fluid drainage.

Contraindications: Congestive heart failure, gastroesophageal reflux, cerebrovascular disease, severe arterial insufficiency.

Props: A blanket and a wall, possibly a pillow.

Avoiding pitfalls: Find the right props for comfort. Use a piece of furniture instead of a wall if it is more comfortable that way.

INSTRUCTIONS:

1. Set a blanket on the floor near a wall or piece of furniture that can support your legs. Lie on one side parallel to the wall.

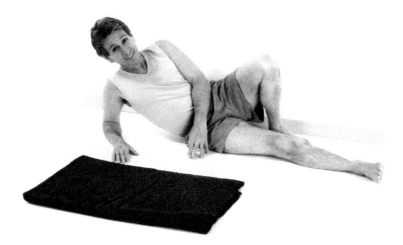

2. Roll over onto your back and raise your legs up the wall. Your legs may be straight or slightly bent. Use a pillow under your head if necessary.

3. Rest. Focus on your breathing: let go of whatever you do not need in this moment.

4. Over one to two months, increase your time in this pose to five to ten minutes.

We recommend this pose for relaxation and assimilation of what you have just learned, but not for sleep.

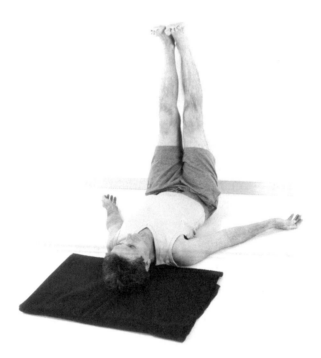

Foot and Ankle *Asana*: Types and Intensity of Movement

Name	Flexion	Extension	Inversion (Supination)	Eversion (Pronation)	Comments
*Tadasana					Finding the four corners
*Standing Lunge with Wall		3	1		Optional toe extension
*Supta Padangusthasana		1		1	Coordination with hips
*Lotus Prep with Wall	2	1		1	Resist the temptation to invert foot
Utkatasana		3		1	Resist the temptation to invert
Uttanasana with Rolled Blanket		3	Balanced[a]	Balanced[a]	Builds arches, lifts metatarsals
*Utthita Parsvakonasana			2		Hip control is critical to foot placement
*Utthita Trikonasana			1		Stretches peroneus longus and brevis
*Prasarita Padottanasana		2	1		Uses foot intrinsics
*Adho Mukha Svanasana		2			Achilles tendon stretch
*Wall Quad	3			1	Plantar flexion
Virasana	3			1	Plantar flexion
Mulabandhasana		2		2	Lateral rotation at ankle
Toe Abduction					Antibunion
Legs up the Wall					Fluid drainage

Note: Poses are graded for the intensity with which they engage the movements in the vertical columns: 1 = a moderate degree; 2 = a substantial degree; 3 = near maximal.

[a]"Balanced" refers to when the muscle groups producing supination and pronation are equal and balance each other.

CHAPTER 14

Scoliosis

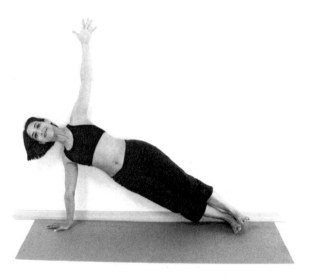

Scoliosis is lateral curvature of the spine. The vertebrae often rotate as well as curve to the side. The rotation is almost invariably toward the convex side and backward, so that the ribs fill up the enlarged space there, producing a bulge or hump in the back. More specific scoliosis diagnoses are made from simple back-to-front X-rays of the neck, chest, and lumbar spine that are then mounted together, yielding a long thin X-ray of the entire spine. There are standard ways of accurately measuring the curves, often with a four- to six-degree margin of error. Curves are generally either simple C-shaped curves or more complex S-shaped ones. The S-shaped curves generally have convex cervical spines and convex thoracolumbar spines in opposite directions. Some scoliosis resolves spontaneously with forward bending and is called idiopathic, meaning "of no known cause." Scoliosis diagnoses are named for the size of the curve, for its place in the spine, and for right (dextro-) or left (levo-) convexity. Thus, the diagno-

sis "thirty-five-degree nonidiopathic rotatory thoracolumbar dextrosco-
liosis" would translate into lay terms as an unchanging thirty-five-
degree curve with its apex on the right, involving the vertebrae of the
chest and abdomen, with a humplike bulge in the right lower back.

In contrast to the other conditions we have discussed so far, scoliosis is rarely painful. Very infrequently, a patient will experience achi-
ness on one side. In young patients, the difficulties are usually
cosmetic, but occasionally it can interfere with childbearing. After a
person with scoliosis has passed age sixty or seventy, though, the scoliosis can become increasingly severe, to the point of limiting breathing.

The causes of scoliosis range from a leg-length discrepancy to partial paralysis, but frequently the cause is unknown. Some believe there
is a hereditary component since it is more common in children of scoli-
otics. It is also more common in women. The standard treatment guide-
lines are "brace patients with curves from twenty to forty degrees,
surgery for those above forty, and expectantly watch those less than
twenty." Deepening of the curve generally drops off dramatically after
the growth spurt at age fifteen to eighteen, but, as already mentioned,
the curvature may progress substantially after middle age.

Despite its ubiquity, there is no convincing evidence that bracing
works. Modern surgical treatment began with insertion of the Harring-
ton rod, a metal dowel to which the vertebral bodies are attached, holding the spine straight as if it were a growing sapling. The most advanced
surgeries as of this writing, the Cotrel-Dubousset and Texas Scottish Rite
Hospital procedures, use extensive wiring to produce a spine that is symmetrical and well formed in three dimensions and gives unending support. But they sacrifice flexibility, and always include the possibility of
complications such as infections, breakdown of the hardware, and aller-
gic reactions, among others. Since the postsurgical spine resembles the
spondyloarthritic one in its immobility, postsurgical patients should see
Chapter 15, on spondyloarthropathies, and pursue the exercises there
that are meant for fused spines. The scoliosis *asana* are not for them.

That there are scoliosis *asana* at all, though, is a recent realization.
We initially began using yoga postures to treat scoliosis out of despera-
tion. One person had ever-increasing scoliosis and was unable to endure
surgical corrections, partially because of limited breathing due to the
scoliosis. We thought at least we could slow the process of further curvature and possibly—just possibly—stop it. After two years of faithful daily

postures, another scoliosis film showed a decrease of the curvature from ninety-three to fifty-three degrees. Then her moderately scoliotic daughter, a yoga teacher as luck would have it, learned the postures and reduced her curve to nearly zero in three months. Since then we have had a number of successes, and one unfortunate but informative episode. A teenager reduced her S-shaped curves from twenty-four and eighteen degrees to twelve and eight degrees with three months of hard and faithful work. Then she got a boyfriend, started smoking, and quit doing yoga. Within three months her curves had returned to twenty-four and eighteen degrees. She is now diligently doing the postures again; perhaps others can learn from this apparent exception.

No one was more surprised than we were when X-rays of people we had been treating actually started to show a reduction in their curves three to six months after beginning the yoga exercises that follow. No one had reported it before. In fact, a number of previous studies had shown that exercise was useless or worse! The old-time exercises that worsened scoliotic curves focused on flexibility. In our clinical practice we made a fresh start. We compared the spine to a tent pole or a radio antenna: These vertical structures are paradoxically held up by forces that are pulling downward. Generally the muscles that perform this same function for our spines apply their forces symmetrically, and the spine is held straight. When the tensions in the muscles, analogous to the guy wires steadying a radio antenna, happen to become asymmetrical, though, the bend of the spine is toward the stronger side, and as it continues, gravity tends to amplify the imbalance. The more flexibility the spine develops, the more gravity and the muscular imbalance are able to bend it! This is why increased flexibility is actually harmful for scoliosis.

There was another key realization: in people with more advanced scoliosis, the ribs tend to migrate backward on the convex (weaker) side. If you examine the back of someone with this condition, the bulging convex side actually looks as though it has the larger muscles. But that is an illusion brought on by the backward migration of the ribs. In reality, the muscles on the concave side are pulling the top and bottom of the spine over toward it. The ribs jut out in the opposite direction, just as the handle of a bow moves away from a taut bowstring.

Our theory is that scoliosis is generally due to asymmetrical weakness of the muscles that support and hold up the spine, and the weakness is on the convex side. Our solution is surprisingly simple: we strengthen

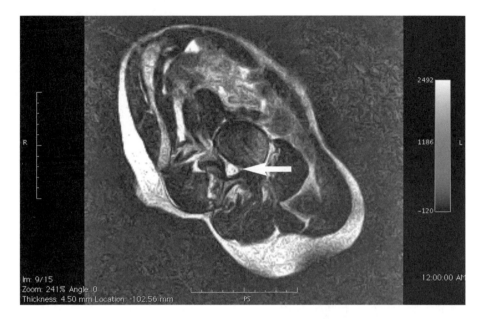

Figure 14. *Spinal stenosis at L4-L5 (MRI). Anatomical position: The central spinal canal is narrowed, placing this person at risk of pain, paresthesias, weakness, and numbness at any point below the narrowing.*

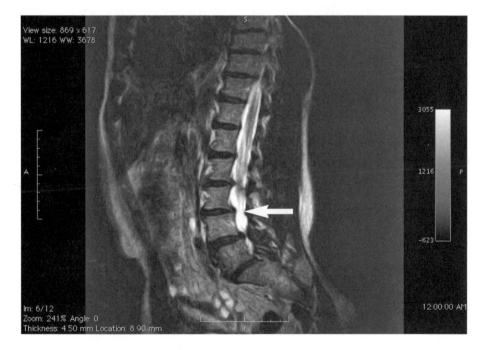

Figure 15. *Spondylolisthesis at L4-L5 (MRI). Standing: Spondylolisthesis occurs when a vertebra slips from its normal alignment, generally forward, drawing the boney perimeter of the spinal canal dangerously close to the nervous tissue within the central canal.*

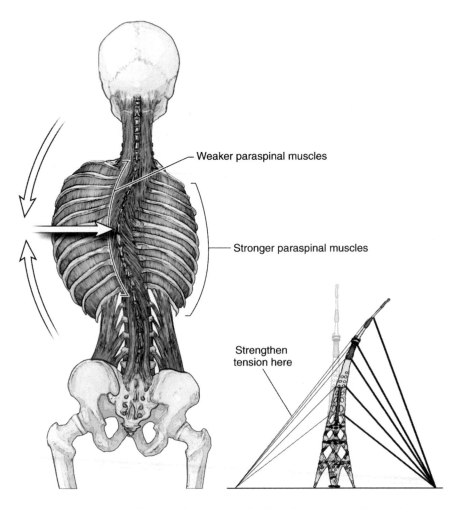

Figure 16. *Correcting scoliosis. The convex side, though appearing larger, is actually the weaker side. Strengthening it brings the spine toward vertical.*

the muscles of the convex side, taking care not to increase the spine's flexibility. The process of strengthening seems to increase the range of motion in exactly the right direction.

Vasisthasana has been one of the most successful poses we have used to reduce and cure scoliosis. It is done asymmetrically, convex-side down. Common sense suggests that it may strengthen muscles on the convex, bulging side, raising that side upward. The images of one of us performing Vasisthasana inside a special MRI machine confirm that the iliopsoas and other vertically oriented muscles actually are put to work asymmetrically during this pose (see pages 267–68).

We cannot stress too strongly that you need to pursue these exercises every single day, with a physician, a yoga therapist, or another person who is skilled enough to help and humble enough to ask questions and obtain scoliosis films every six months.

Part I: Getting to Know Your Curve

Important Note: The first four poses are for learning more about the nature, size, direction, rotation, and malleability of your curve. You will do better if you first understand what is going on in your back. These Part I exercises will not lessen your curve. Do these poses possibly every month to note any changes. Do *not* do them every day: increasing flexibility will *worsen* your curve, not cure it.

---

1. TADASANA WITH SIDE BEND (Mountain Pose)

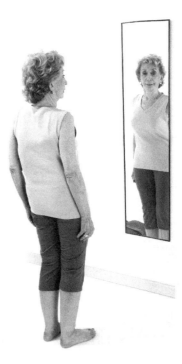

Purpose: To understand your particular spinal curves.

Contraindications: Plantar fasciitis, balance disorder.

Prop: A mirror.

Avoiding pitfalls: Keep your legs firm for good balance. Be patient as you observe your own movements as objectively as possible.

INSTRUCTIONS:

1. Stand facing a mirror with your feet hip-width apart. Wear clothes that are tight enough to reveal your body's contours. See where your body is asymmetrical. Is one shoulder higher? (This side is probably your convex side in the thoracic spine.) Is one hip protruding? (This may be your concave side in the lumbar

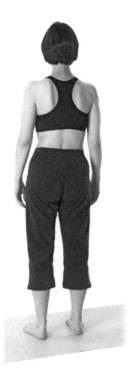

spine.) Is one side of the ribs protruding? (This is probably your convex side in the thoracic spine.) Is one hip higher? (This side is probably your concave side in the lumbar spine.)

2. Firm your legs, take a big breath in, and raise your arms up overhead. Interlace your fingers over your head, palms up.

3. Exhale as you lean to the right and observe how your spine moves. Does it feel restricted in the upper part or the lower part? It will be more difficult to lean toward the convex side, and easier to lean toward the concave side. Does your back want to turn as you do this? A rotatory element in the scoliosis will cause a turn as you bend to the side.

4. Return to center, and repeat on the other side.

5. Write down what you discover about your curve, and confirm it with another observer.

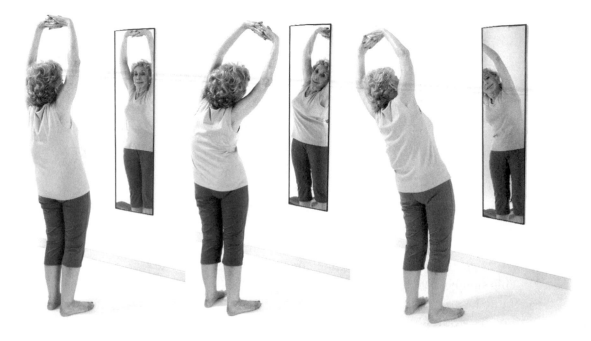

2. SIDE CHILD SPINE

Purpose: To understand your particular spinal curves.

Contraindications: Meniscal tear, prepatellar bursitis, rotator cuff tear.

Props: A yoga mat and a blanket.

Avoiding pitfalls: Use padding under and just below your knees. Position the hips over the knees. Keep your arms plugged into your shoulder sockets.

INSTRUCTIONS:

1. Come down onto your hands and knees on the blanket.
2. Walk your hands to the right, bend your right arm, and position your right forearm to support your forehead. Extend your left arm forward at an angle toward the right that begins to stretch your left side.
3. Firm your arm muscles. Lift up the side ribs and armpit. Pull the arm into the shoulder joint, connecting the whole left side.
4. Extend back with your left hip, and reach out through the left hand, making a long continuous arc of stretch along your left side.
5. Repeat on the other side.
6. Observe which area of your back bends easily this way, and which part does not. Note the distribution of air as you inhale.

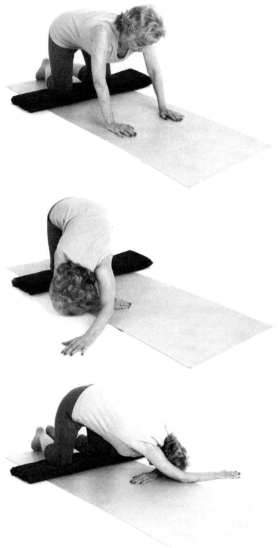

3. EXPLORATORY PRASARITA PADOTTANASANA

Purpose: To understand your spinal curves when reversing gravitational influence.

Contraindications: Balance disorder, wet macular degeneration, cerebrovascular disease, Chiari malformation, vasovagal episodes.

Props: A yoga mat, possibly a block.

Avoiding pitfalls: Spread your feet wide enough apart so your pelvis moves easily. Place the feet parallel to protect your knees.

INSTRUCTIONS:

1. Place your feet four to five feet apart. When you stretch your arms out to the side, your wrists should be over your ankles. This is a good way to determine the width of your stance, based on your body's proportions. Do the best you can.
2. Make sure that your feet are parallel, both facing forward.
3. Firm your leg muscles, hugging the bones from all sides.
4. Gather your strength up into the core of the pelvis, and maintain this throughout the pose.
5. Hold your feet and shins firmly toward the midline and, challenging that, push both thighs apart without rotating them. Imagine that you

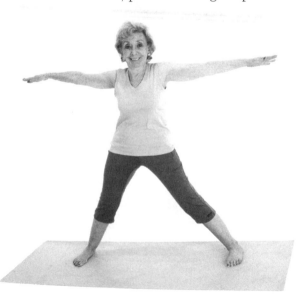

are riding a very large horse, and you have to widen your thighs to straddle it, but you also need to hold on.
6. Curl your tailbone down and lift your abdomen up.
7. Keep your legs firm. Extend your energy down through your legs to the floor, rooting yourself for stability.
8. Inhale, extend your spine up, and while exhaling, bend straight forward to touch the floor or a block.

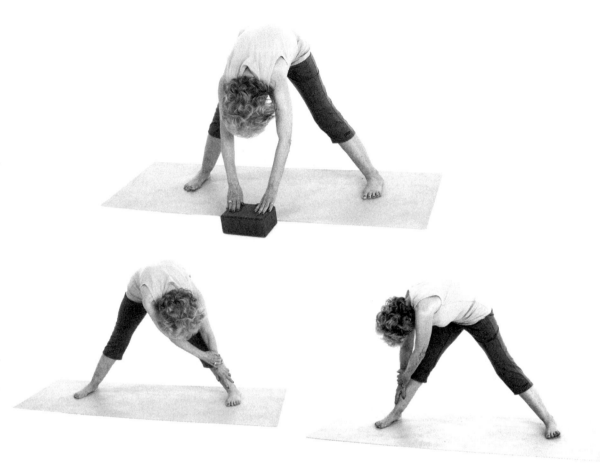

9. Playfully but cautiously move your torso in this hanging position. Experiment with lateral and rotating movements; try to understand your curve. See which kinds of movements are easy, and to which there is resistance. See if this matches what you discovered in the previous exercises.

10. You can walk your hands toward the right and left—again to gain information, not to stretch anything.

11. To come up: Place your hands on your hips, step your feet a bit closer together, and pull your shoulders back. Then inhale smoothly as you raise your torso to vertical.

4. WALL DOG/TABLE DOG

Purpose: To understand your spinal curves.

Contraindications: Rotator cuff and shoulder impingement syndromes, spondylolisthesis.

Prop: A wall or a table.

Avoiding pitfalls: Choose a height for your arms that is comfortable, one that allows you to stay in the pose long enough to make observations. Use the wall if you are stiffer, the table if you are more limber.

INSTRUCTIONS:

1. Stand near a wall or tabletop with your feet hip-width apart and parallel.
2. Place your hands on the wall or tabletop, shoulder-width apart and parallel. Rotate the upper arms so that the biceps face up. Straighten your elbows.

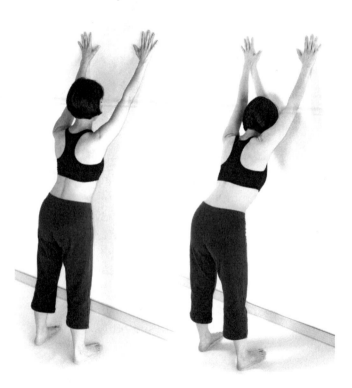

3. With your arms and legs firm, and your chest soft, bend forward with your upper body, reaching your hips back. Bend your knees.
4. Widen your sitting bones and thighs. This will create a slight arch in your lower back.
5. Firm your abdominal muscles and lengthen through the lower part of the spine without eliminating the arch.
6. Straighten your knees as much as possible.
7. Extend fully from your pelvis in two directions: out through your spine and

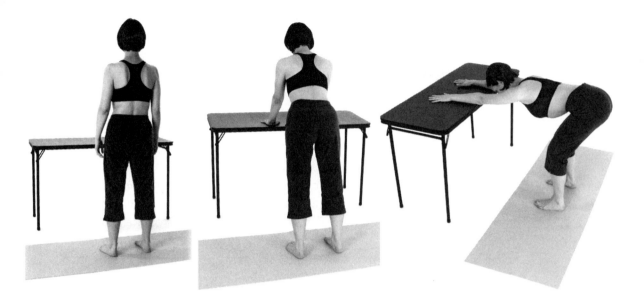

arms, and down through your legs. This energetic lengthening will help you to know where your body is more mobile and less mobile.

8. Look for the following (ideally with someone else watching to report what he or she sees). What you see will help you determine where your curves are, and therefore help you to do the exercises on the correct side:

- If one shoulder is higher, if one arm is difficult to straighten, or if the ribs are more prominent on one side, that is the convex side of your thoracic spine.
- If one side of the waistline looks more indented or if one hip is harder to stretch away from the wall, that is your concave side in the lumbar spine.

9. Compare these observations with those you made in previous poses.
10. To come up, breathe in and step toward the wall or table as you raise your torso.

Part II: Strengthening the Convex Side

Important Note: These are the exercises to do every day. The more you do them, the sooner you will begin to reduce your curve and approach true symmetry. Many poses are described in several stages, which allows you to choose the level of challenge that suits you. We recommend that you begin with Stage I, and if it is quite easy, progress through the stages until you find the one that is moderately challenging for you. Stay with that stage for a few weeks or so, and when it becomes too easy, move on to the next stage. It is nearly indispensable to have a yoga therapist, physician, or physical therapist to help with positioning and to check you at least monthly to be sure that the correct muscles are actually doing the right thing. You should obtain scoliosis X-rays every six months to measure your progress. A change of more than six degrees is meaningful.

1. SEATED CRESCENT LEVELER

Purpose: To use strength and leverage to bring the spine more into balance, and to strengthen the muscles that do so.

Contraindications: Anterior labral tear, herniated lumbar disc, recent vertebral fracture.

Prop: A chair.

Avoiding pitfalls: Follow instructions to level the pelvis, then integrate the force you apply with your arms throughout your torso to assist in leveling the rest of the spine.

INSTRUCTIONS:

1. Sit sideways on a straight chair, with your concave side away from the chair back, whether it is the lumbar or the cervicothoracic part of your spine. Place one hand on the back of the chair, the other on your thigh.

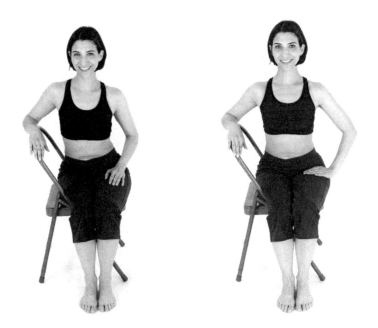

2. (a) If it is your lower back you want to level: Carefully push on the chair back and push down the hip that is higher. Your waist and lower abdomen will move away from the chair back and you will reduce the rotation slightly. (b) If it is your upper back or neck: Carefully push on the chair back to move your ribs and upper spine away from the chair. The same derotation will occur here also.

3. In both cases, attempt to equalize the length of both sides of your body, from your shoulders to your hips. Breathe and hold the pose for ten to twenty seconds for the first few weeks, then for as long as possible.

4. Feel internally for the midline!

5. If you have a complex curve, in which there are two convex parts— one lower down, one higher up—instruction 2(a) will need to be done on one side, and 2(b) on the other. Do not repeat either 2(a) or 2(b) for the concave sides.

2. RESISTED ABDUCTION OF ARM (one side only)

Purpose: To strengthen the paraspinal and related muscles on the convex side.

Contraindication: Balance disorder.

Prop: A wall.

Avoiding pitfalls: Do not let the trunk move toward or away from the wall.

INSTRUCTIONS:

1. Stand with your concave side toward the wall, your arm by your side and the back of your hand against the wall.
2. Place your feet hip-width apart, with your leg muscles engaged, in your best Tadasana alignment.
3. Press your hand into the wall.
4. At first, *let* the rest of your body move in response.
5. Continue pressing *without* letting the rest of your body move in

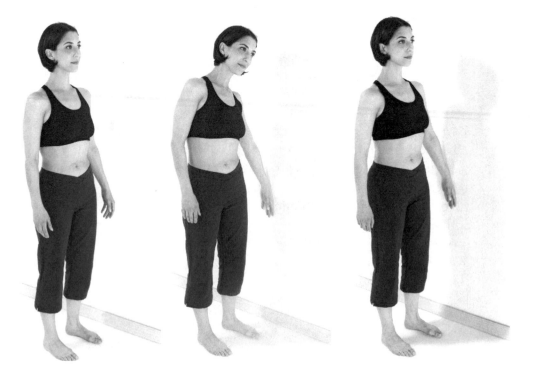

response. You should be using the muscles on the side away from the wall to stay steady and still.

6. Do this until the muscles on the side away from the wall feel tired. This may take anywhere from thirty seconds to five minutes or longer.

7. It takes practice to avoid leaning into or away from the wall. At first push gently. After a few weeks, using greater pressure against the wall will reduce the amount of time it takes to get tired. You are building muscle strength here.

---

3. VASISTHASANA (four stages)

Purpose: To strengthen the paraspinal and other muscles of the convex side.

Contraindications: Profound weakness, Hill-Sachs deformity, balance disorder, carpal tunnel syndrome at wrist on convex side.

Props: A wall, a yoga mat, a block, and a chair.

Avoiding pitfalls: Pull your upper arm and shoulder back before putting weight on it. Line your head up with your spine. Don't be tentative: be firm and expansive with your whole body. Note: This is an extremely versitile pose, as pages 267–68 indicate.

INSTRUCTIONS:

Preparation for Stages I and II

1. Lie on a yoga mat on the floor, with your convex side down.
2. Rest on your forearm, with your body lined up parallel to the wall and your knees bent. Pull your shoulders back.
3. Let the side of your ribs sag down toward the floor.

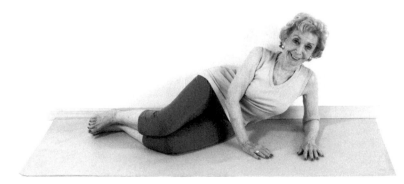

Stage I

4. Inhaling, firm your muscles (especially arms and abdomen). Lift the side of your ribs up away from the floor. Let your hips and legs remain on the floor. Press on a block (if needed) with your upper hand.
5. Hold the side of your ribs up until your back feels tired on the convex side.
6. Slowly release.

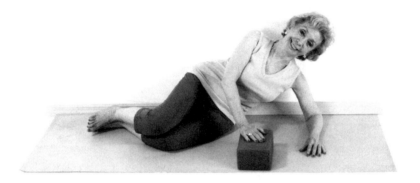

Stage II

1. Complete instructions 1 through 4 above. When you lift, as per instruction 4, lift your hips up as well, so that only your calves, ankles, and feet remain on the floor.

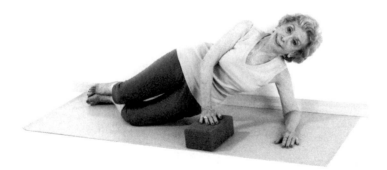

Stage III

1. Complete instructions 1 through 3 under Preparation for Stages I and II.
2. Extend your legs straight out.
3. Place one foot on top of the other. Pull the little-toe edge of the top foot up toward the outer ankle bone.
4. Lift your whole body up, from ribs to ankles.

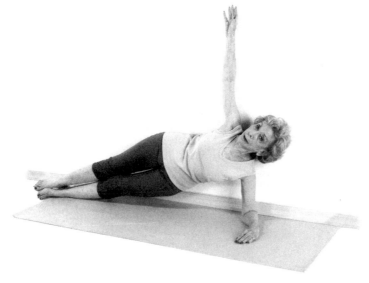

Stage IV

Go into the pose from the Adho Mukha Svanasana Pose (see page 66) as follows:

1. Place a chair next to your mat in case you need it for support.
2. Perform Adho Mukha Svanasana, the Full Downward Dog Pose.

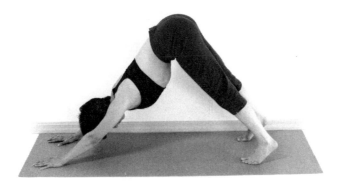

3. From the Full Downward Dog Pose, shift your weight onto the out-side of your foot on the convex side of your scoliosis.

4. Reposition the hand on the convex side, lining it up with the foot, the fingers angled outward slightly.

5. Firm the upper arm and pull the shoulder back.

6. Revolve over onto the arm on the convex side and the outer edge of the foot on the convex side until your back is parallel to the wall.

7. Use your upper hand on the chair for balance if you need it. One option here (not pictured) is to place the upper foot at midmat for additional aid in balance. Otherwise, stretch your arm up along the wall.

8. Raise your ribs and hips high enough to make one long diagonal line from head to feet.

9. Breathe with a bright energy throughout your whole body.

10. Remain until the convex side tires.

11. Return to the Full Downward Dog Pose, followed by the Child's Pose (see page 92).

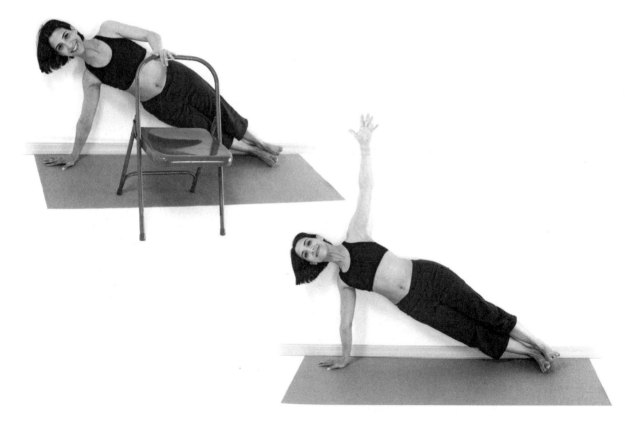

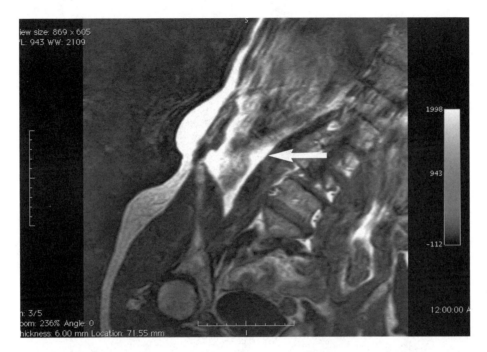

Figure 17. *(MRI). Vasisthasana with scoliosis, convex side down. Asymmetrical tightening of the iliopsoas muscle on the convex side strengthens this muscle, effectively reestablishing symmetrical forces on the spine, reducing the scoliosis.*

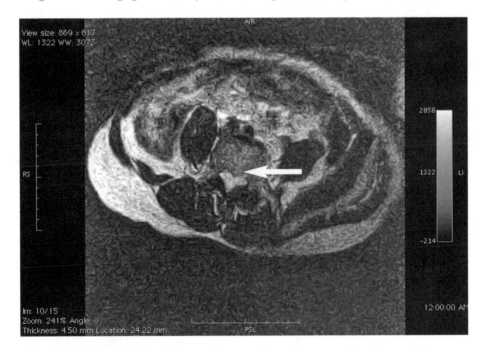

Figure 18. *Vasisthasana (MRI). The central canal is broadened, reassuming its normal heart-shaped form. No study confirms that Vasisthasana gives lasting benefit to people with spinal stenosis. However, this image suggests that it is safe.*

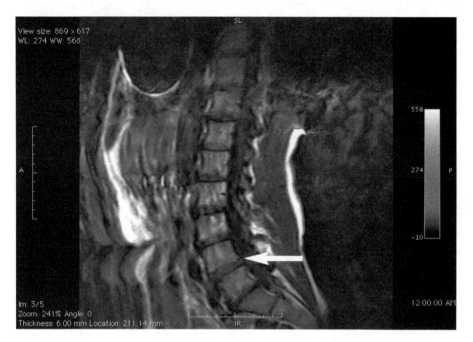

Figure 19. *Vasisthasana (MRI). Spondylolisthesis is also effectively countered in Vasisthasana. Like spinal stenosis, no definitive study verifies a lasting benefit at this point, but the possibilities of treating these serious and often surgical conditions are intriguing.*

4. ANANTASANA (two stages)

Purpose: To straighten simple and complex curves.

Contraindication: Profound weakness.

Props: A wall, a mat, and a belt.

Avoiding pitfalls: Stay lined up with the wall as much as possible.

INSTRUCTIONS:

Preparations for Both Stages

1. Lie on the side of the thoracic convexity, with padding placed under your side and with your back against a wall. Bend your legs slightly. Extend your lower arm out along the wall, and prop your head up with your hand.

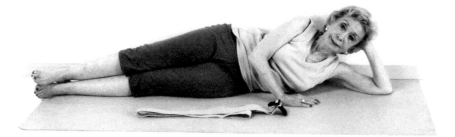

2. Place your upper hand in front of you on the floor to help with balance. Have a belt handy for Stage II.

Stage I

3. Lift the underside of your ribs up off the floor.
4. Pull your lower arm in toward you. Slowly continue until the forearm is vertical, or as close as you can get to it. You may experience only the pull, without any movement of the arm taking place.
5. Stay in your best approximation of the pose for as long as you can, in order to strengthen the convex side.

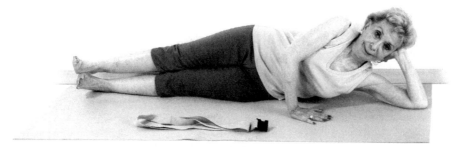

Stage II

6. Bend your upper leg, hold your toe or hook the belt onto the foot, and turn the heel forward to rotate the leg outward.
7. Stretch the leg upward.

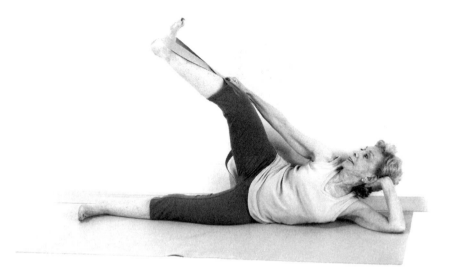

8. Straighten the knee as much as possible. Keep your back against the wall and use your abdominal and back muscles to stabilize your pelvis as you raise the extended leg. You can gaze up or forward. Raise your ribs away from the floor as well. Don't forget to breathe!

9. Release down and rest on your back.

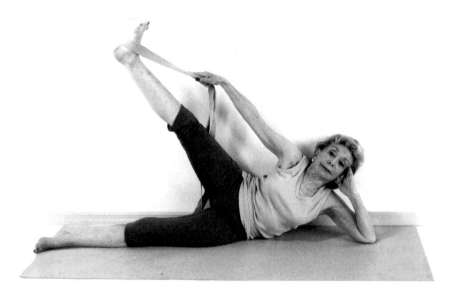

5. ARDHA SALABHASANA VARIATION

Purpose: To strengthen the relevant spinal muscles in simple and complex curves. This pose is effective when the arm on the side of the convex upper curve is raised. It also strengthens the lumbar musculature on the opposite side.

Contraindications: Extreme hypertension, lumbar spinal stenosis.

Props: A yoga mat and a blanket for comfort.

Avoiding pitfalls: If you have a complex curve involving the left lumbar and right thoracocervical spine, then lift the right arm and leg. Lift the left arm and leg if the curve involves the right lumbar and left thoracocervical spine.

Breathe continuously, elongate your neck and tailbone; retract your shoulders. Fully engage your legs. Carefully balance between pulling in and stretching out, which happen simultaneously when you are in the pose.

INSTRUCTIONS:

1. Lie facedown on a mat. Place your forehead on the floor and extend your arms out alongside your ears, palms facing in. If this starting position is uncomfortable for your lower back, neck, or shoulders, put a folded blanket or pillow under your chest and pelvis.
2. Firm your arm, leg, and spinal muscles, drawing into your core of strength. Widen your thighs, making space for the tailbone to curl downward. Stretch back through your legs all the way to the toes, being careful not to squeeze your buttock muscles toward each other, but press the whole pelvis down.

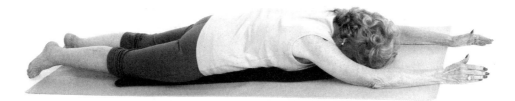

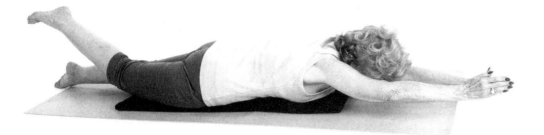

3. Inhale, lift, and extend through one arm and leg on the same side. (See "Avoiding pitfalls" above to determine which side you use.)
4. Wholeheartedly lengthen through your entire body.
5. Remain in the pose until you are tired, then rest down onto the floor.

---

6. JATHARA PARIVARTANASANA (variation with chair)

Purpose: To use the thighs to help balance the pelvis and lower back.

Contraindications: Inguinal or abdominal hernia, spondylolisthesis.

Props: A yoga mat and a chair, possibly a blanket or pillow.

Avoiding pitfalls: Pad yourself as needed, perhaps with a pillow placed under the side of your ribs, and a larger support under your head to rest it comfortably.

INSTRUCTIONS:

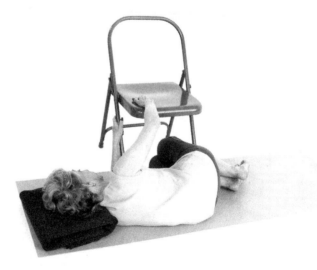

1. Lie on your convex side (in this description it is your left side) and bend your knees up toward your chest so they will fit under the seat of a straight chair. Support the chair with your hands.
2. Breathe and open your thighs

away from each other. Widen your sitting bones as well. Your left leg will push against the floor and your right leg will push against the underside of the chair seat. Do this action strongly enough to lift your left ribs slightly off the floor.

3. As you maintain the position, breathe and make more space inside.
4. Take it into a twist: steady the chair with your left hand, and rest your right hand on your waistline. Curl your right shoulder back and down toward the floor, twisting your upper back to the right.
5. Stay with that stretch for several breaths, then free your legs, unwind, and roll onto your back to rest.

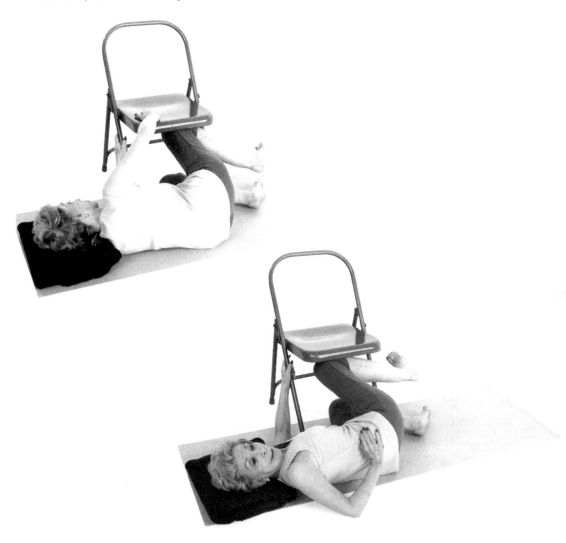

CHAPTER 15

Ankylosing Spondylitis

Spondyloarthropathies are different from any of the other conditions we treat in this book. Other types of arthritis and scoliosis can occur to different degrees on a continuum, and the poses offered for them can be practiced at varying levels of intensity. But spondyloarthropathies progress slowly until there is a point of no return. Similar to water slowly getting colder and colder and then suddenly turning to ice, the very nature of the joint changes—it is not deformed or inflamed but

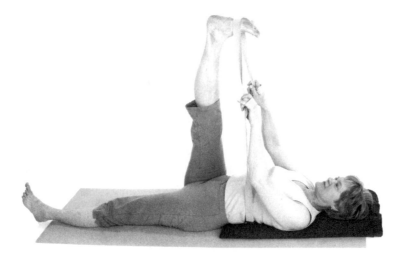

rather becomes frozen. Motion at that point is impossible. The causes, as we saw in Chapter 1, are autoimmune issues, reactions to infection, and genetic factors. People with spondyloarthropathies whose spine has not yet fused are treated one way; those whose spines are no longer mobile are treated another.

The strategy for unfused spines is to keep the vertebral joints in active motion daily, to prevent or at least delay the fusion at the joint by breaking up any adhesions between the bones to keep them moving independently. The thoracic spine-rib joints and the vertebra-vertebra joints generally fuse in the late teens to early twenties, so this work must begin early.

If fusion has already taken place, and we have a so-called bamboo spine, the goal is to increase the range of motion of the hips and shoulders in order to maximize their function without damaging the cervical spine, lumbosacral spine, or sacroiliac joints. This extremely worthy but delicate work demands perceptive and experienced guidance. *Do not*

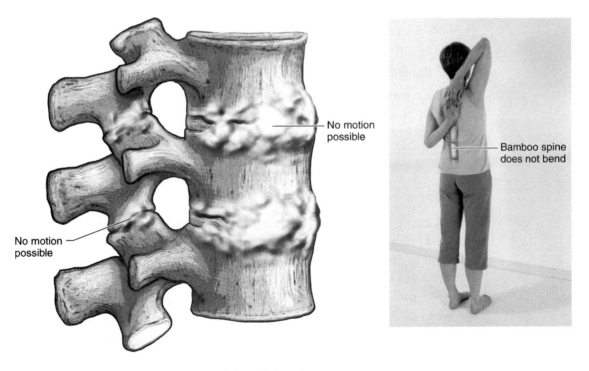

Figure 20. *The fused segments of the ankylosed spine.*

think that you can "convert" a fused spine to an unfused spine by doing exercises for the unfused spine. You will very likely hurt yourself.

Caution: If you are unsure whether your spine has fused or not, do not guess. If your spine is partially fused (only some vertebrae adhere together), for safety's sake it should be treated as a fused spine. Simple X-rays and a visit to your physician should clarify the matter. It is critical to determine this in order to select the exercises that will be best for you.

Ankylosing Spondylitis: Poses for People Whose Spines Are Already Fused

1. ARMS CLASPED BEHIND (variation of Salabhasana)

Purpose: To strengthen the extensors of the shoulders and stretch the flexors.

Contraindications: Recent rotator cuff tear. If you have carpal tunnel syndrome, use a belt.

Prop: Possibly a belt.

Avoiding pitfalls: Be sure to lift up your chest and spine before you pull your upper arms back. Do not lock your elbows, and if your back arches a lot, pull back through the sides of your waistline.

INSTRUCTIONS:

1. Stand tall, with feet parallel and hip-width apart, and your hands clasped behind you or your wrists inside a looped belt.
2. Breathe in and lift the front of your chest so that your shoulders are square across from side to side, and not slumped down on the edges.
3. Strongly pull your upper arms back, rotate them outward, and push outward against the resistance of your hand clasp or the belt. Bending your elbows slightly will help move the upper arms back correctly.

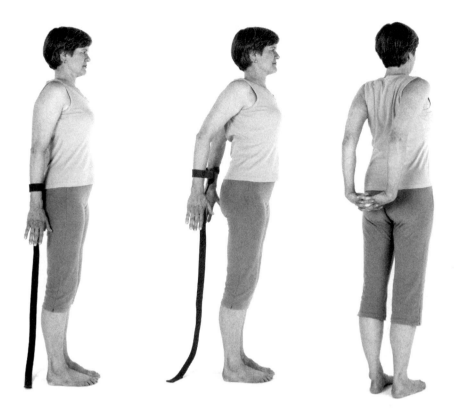

4. The shoulder blades will move back, together, and down. If your ribs go forward, pull back through your waistline to restrain the movement.

5. Hold the pose for a few breaths. Do so vigorously. Expand from your center.

2. STRAP HANGER

Purpose: To maintain and increase the range of motion in shoulder abduction.

Contraindication: Rotator cuff syndrome.

Prop: A wall.

Avoiding pitfalls: Keep your body oriented perpendicular to the wall.

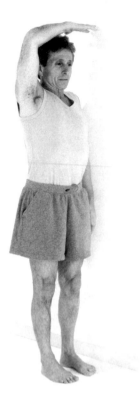

INSTRUCTIONS:

1. Stand with your left shoulder touching the wall.
2. Inhale and begin to raise your right arm out to the side, with your palm facing upward.
3. Continue moving the arm up and overhead until you touch the wall. At this point your palm will face downward.
4. Exhaling, bring your arm down and rest.
5. Repeat several times on one side, with fluid movement supported by your breath.
6. Repeat on the other side.

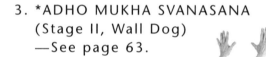

3. *ADHO MUKHA SVANASANA (Stage II, Wall Dog) —See page 63.

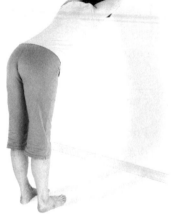

This pose gives the torso a gentle stretch without bending the spine.

4. FROG

Purpose: To stretch and strengthen the hips and legs.

Contraindications: Moderate or severe anterior cruciate or meniscal tears, chondromalacia patellae, profound weakness.

Prop: A wall.

Avoiding pitfalls: Keep your knees facing out over your toes.

INSTRUCTIONS:

1. Stand with your back to the wall, legs turned out forty-five degrees to the side.
2. Inhale and lift your spine.
3. Bend your knees until your thighs are parallel to the floor. The knees should point in the same direction as the toes.
4. Place your hands over the tops of your thighs, near the hips, with your fingers pointing outward.
5. Press down with your hands, allowing you to lift your spine up more and curl your tailbone down. You can lean slightly forward if that feels right.

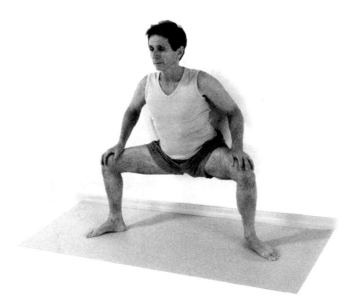

6. Widen your shoulders as you pull your elbows to the sides.
7. Hold with constant strength.
8. When you are ready to come up, push down through your feet and straighten your legs up, releasing your hands.

5. PRASARITA PADOTTANASANA WITH TABLE

Purpose: To stretch the hips and shoulders and mobilize the spine as a unit.

Contraindications: Genu valgum (knock-knees), ischial bursitis.

Prop: A table or a desk.

Avoiding pitfalls: If you feel strain in your shoulders or arms, place your elbows on the table, shoulder-width apart, instead of your hands.

INSTRUCTIONS:

1. Stand facing a table or desk, two to three feet away from it, with your feet four to five feet apart and your hands on your hips.
2. Inhaling, lift your spine up and tone your leg muscles.
3. Exhale. Bend forward from your hips. Place your hands on the table-top, shoulder-width apart.

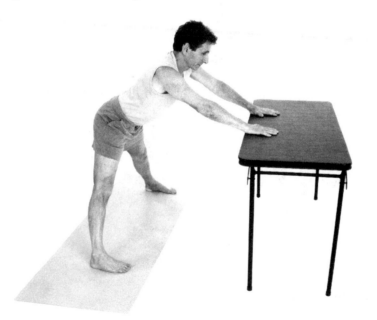

4. On your next exhalation, slide your hands forward enough so that your back comes down parallel with the tabletop. Bend your knees to help your pelvis to tilt, with the sitting bones pointing back and up, and the top of the sacrum down.

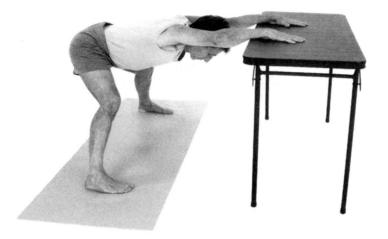

5. Lift your arms and armpits up away toward the ceiling as much as possible while your hands are still on the table.
6. Stretch your sitting bones back and apart. Straighten your knees as much as possible.

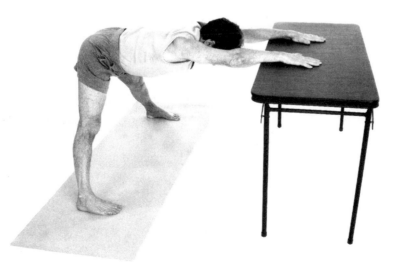

7. Firm your abdomen and let the middle of your back respond to the pull of gravity, softening down, but without strain.

8. Keep full power in your legs and arms while in the pose, breathing steadily.

9. When you are ready to come up, walk toward the table.

---

6. GARUDASANA ARMS ONLY

Purpose: To improve shoulder mobility by stretching the superior two-thirds of the trapezius, rhomboids, deltoids, and teres minor.

Contraindications: Labral tears, Hill-Sachs deformity.

Prop: A chair.

Avoiding pitfalls: Do not force the pose. If it is too difficult, do the Crossover Cactus in the shoulder series (see page 105).

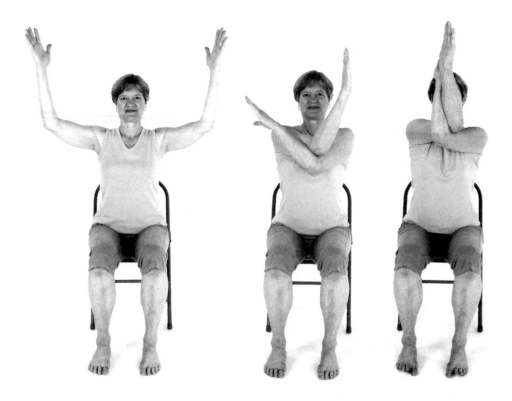

INSTRUCTIONS:

1. Sit toward the front of the chair, with your spine tall and feet flat.
2. Pull your sitting bones and buttocks back and apart with your hands.
3. Bring your arms in front of you, bending the elbows at ninety degrees. Point your hands upward.
4. Hook your right elbow or at least the forearm under your left elbow crease.
5. Intertwine your forearms so that the fingers of your left hand hook onto the palm of your right hand.
6. Inhaling, lift from inside your chest, and pull your upper arms back into your shoulder sockets.
7. On your next inhalation, lift your elbows up, keeping your hands pointing straight up. On exhalation, slide your shoulder blades gently down your back.
8. Hold with equanimity for several breaths, then release and do the other side.

---

7. GOMUKHASANA ARMS ONLY

Purpose: To stretch the pectoralis, latissimus dorsi, teres major, subscapularis, deltoid, and triceps.

Contraindications: Acromioclavicular subluxation, posterior labral tear.

Prop: A belt.

Avoiding pitfalls: Stand up tall to avoid distorting the spine.

INSTRUCTIONS:

1. Stand in neutral Tadasana (see page 59), with your feet hip-width apart. Lift up from within (Inner Body Bright, see Appendix III) so that the sides of your body are long and your collarbones are square across.
2. Place a belt over one shoulder.
3. Raise your right arm in front of you. Turn the palm up.

4. Retract the arm back into the socket and raise it up near your ear.

5. Bend the elbow so your fingers can reach down by the back of your neck. This hand will grasp either the belt or your other hand, which will come back and up. If you do not expect to be able to clasp your hands together, hold the belt with your right hand now. Then bring your left arm out to the side, turn your thumb down, and keep the hand stable as you pull the upper left arm back into its socket.

6. Bend your left arm in with the palm facing out. Reach up between your shoulder blades. Hook your fingers to catch the fingers of the right hand, or hold the belt.

7. Now that you have got the basic shape, it is time to check yourself: Did you bend sideways? Do your ribs jut forward? Is your right arm as vertical as possible? The most difficult part is to get that bottom arm in toward the midline and up. Work patiently.

8. Hold the pose for a few breaths.

9. Gently release, then reverse the arms and repeat as above.

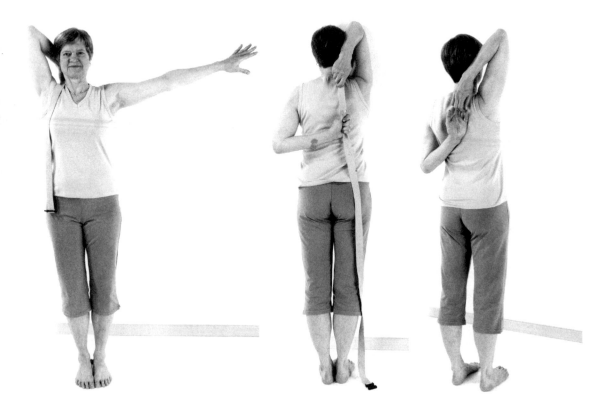

10. You can lean the upper elbow against a wall for support, which takes some of the strain out of the pose. Maintain the core strength of your torso to avoid arching your back. Let the wall work to increase the range of motion of your shoulder.

11. In this somewhat constricting pose, work toward expanding from the inside.

---

8. SITTING LUNGE WITH CHAIR

Purpose: To give a strong, supported stretch to the rectus femoris, iliopsoas, and the adductor group.

Contraindications: Ischial bursitis, medial or lateral meniscal or anterior or posterior cruciate tear, knee effusion.

Prop: A chair.

Avoid pitfalls: As in all hip extension movements, when the leg goes back, the lower back may arch too much. Work into it, and contract and lift your abdominal muscles the whole time to support the lower back.

INSTRUCTIONS:

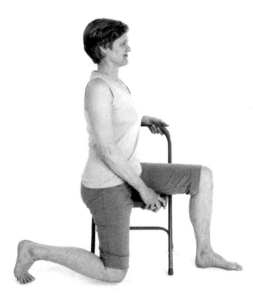

1. Sit sideways on the front edge of a chair, with your left thigh fully supported by the chair seat and your right leg hanging straight down off the front edge.

2. Lean forward and use your hands on the chair as needed for stability.

3. Firm all the leg muscles, and widen your buttocks and thighs, as in the Pressure Cooker (see page 73).

4. Lengthen your tailbone down and lift your abdominal muscles up to stabilize your pelvis. Resting your hand on your hip

will remind you to keep the pelvis as vertical as possible.

5. Once steady, carefully inch your right leg back behind you. The knee will remain bent as the thigh moves farther from vertical.

6. Breathe deeply as you reach back through the back leg; find the appropriate level of intensity of effort.

7. Stretch your leg back maximally, if possible, until the knee is straight.

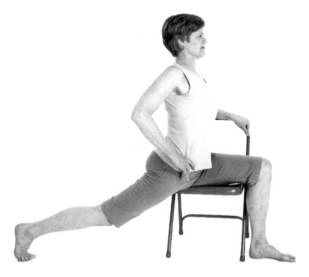

8. Lift your torso up to vertical, using the support of the chair.

9. Enjoy this deep hip stretch, made safe by the support of the chair.

10. Bring the back leg forward to change sides.

---

9. *WINDSHIELD WIPER—See page 80.

This pose can be done in bed. It is not necessary to get onto the floor.

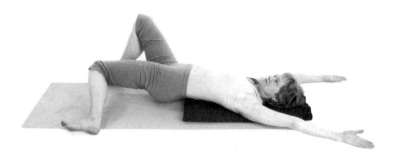

In this pose the hip rotates inward toward the midline and the side of the body elongates with minimal spinal movement.

10. *SUPTA PADANGUSTHASANA—See page 83.

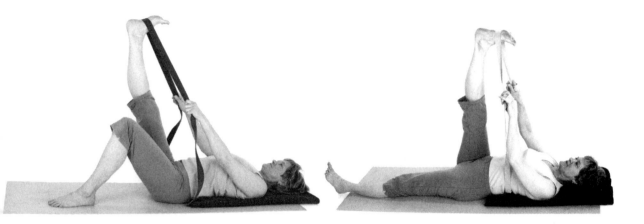

This basic leg stretch ensures a healthy freedom in the hips so that everyday movements do not jar the spine.

Ankylosing Spondylitis: Poses for People Whose Spines Are Still Unfused

1. *WINDSHIELD WIPER—See page 80.

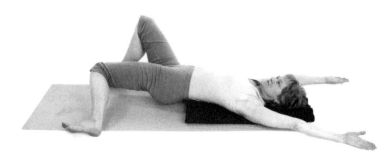

Lengthen the sides of the body before back bending with this warm-up pose.

2. *BHUJANGASANA—See page 89.

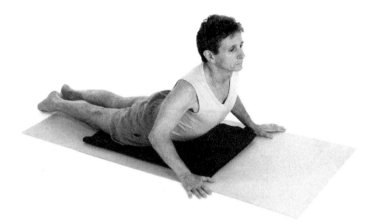

This back bend builds strength in the upper back, shoulders, and arms, while bringing safe cervical and thoracic vertebral motion.

3. SALABHASANA

Purpose: To strengthen back extensors, move all vertebrae.

Contraindications: Colostomy, spinal stenosis, anterior labral tear or SLAP lesion.

Props: A yoga mat, a folded blanket, and a belt.

Avoiding pitfalls: Come up into the pose slowly and with care to avoid a sudden extreme load on your neck or lower back.

INSTRUCTIONS:

1. Lie on your stomach on a mat, with the folded blanket placed under your abdomen and your pubic bone on the mat. This will help to prevent lower back strain.
2. Hold a looped belt in one hand, stretch your arms in parallel behind your back, and loop the belt around both wrists.

3. With your forehead on the floor, roll your shoulders back (up toward the ceiling) and lengthen the sides of your body between your hips and your arms.

4. Firm your legs and lengthen your tailbone, firming your buttocks without squeezing them together.

5. Inhaling, lift your arms, pushing out against the belt.

6. Lift your head and legs, stretching your legs back as they rise.

7. Pull forward through your chest to lengthen the spine as it rises.

8. Stay up for several breaths, making your body as buoyant as possible.

9. Release back to the floor and remove the belt.

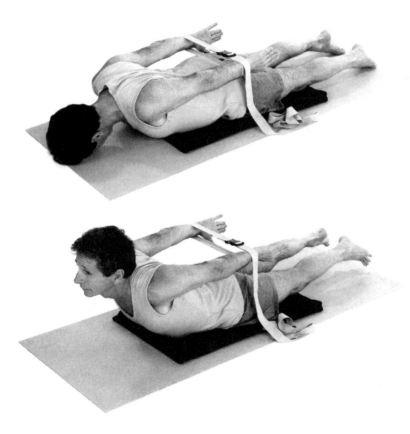

4. *CHILD'S POSE—See page 92.

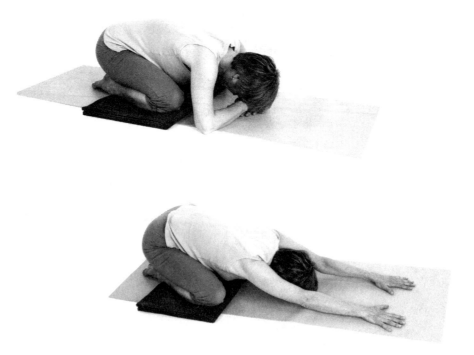

This resting pose should follow the back bends you have just done.

5. GOMUKHASANA (Full Cow Pose)

Purpose: To stretch the hip abductors and shoulder flexors and extensors, and move rib-sternal connections.

Contraindications: Absolute: total hip replacement. Relative: knee tightness, instability, or previous injury; ischial bursitis.

Props: A mat, one or two folded blankets, and a belt.

Avoiding pitfalls: If this pose is a challenge, practice the arms and legs separately first (see pages 283 and 127). Use enough height under your hips to sit up straight with your pelvis vertical, not sloping back.

INSTRUCTIONS:

1. Place the folded blankets on the mat, with one corner pointing forward.
2. Sit on the front corner of the blankets as shown, with your left knee pointing forward and your right knee up.
3. Grasp your right leg with both hands and cross it over the left.
4. Stack your right knee on top of your left, with the feet to the sides.
5. If your knees stay very high up, use more support under your hips.
6. Manually separate the buttocks as much as possible. This will free your pelvis to bend forward.
7. Inhale, lift through your spine, and tone the leg muscles.
8. Place the belt over your right shoulder in case you need it to connect your hands.
9. Raise your right arm up in front of you at a forty-five-degree angle, turn your palm up, and retract the arm into the shoulder socket.
10. Fully stretch your arm up beside your head and bend your elbow, the hand coming behind your head. Grasp the belt or reach your fingers down.

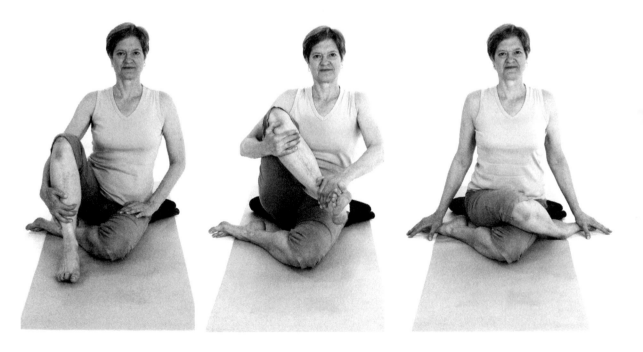

11. Bring your left arm to the side, thumb down, and move the very top of the arm back any amount you can. You will feel your shoulder blade slide toward the spine as you do this.
12. Reach your left arm up behind your back and grasp the belt or your other hand.
13. Lift and widen the front of your chest and look straight ahead.
14. Be as content and centered as possible as you maintain the pose.
15. Release. Repeat on the other side.

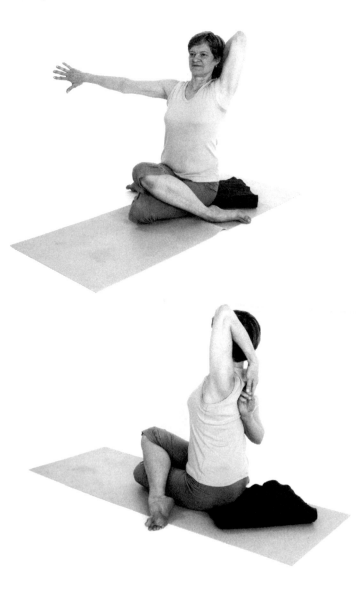

6. GARUDASANA ARMS ONLY

Purpose: To produce a strong shoulder stretch that addresses the superior two-thirds of the trapezius, rhomboids, deltoids, and teres minor. To move the ribs' spinal joints.

Contraindications: Posterior labral tear, Hill-Sachs deformity.

Prop: A chair (optional).

Avoiding pitfalls: Do not force it. If this is too difficult, do the Crossover Cactus (see page 105) from the shoulder series.

INSTRUCTIONS:

1. Sit toward the front of the chair, with your spine tall and feet flat.
2. Pull your sitting bones and buttocks back and apart with your hands.
3. Bring your arms in front of you, bend the elbows at ninety degrees, and point your hands up.

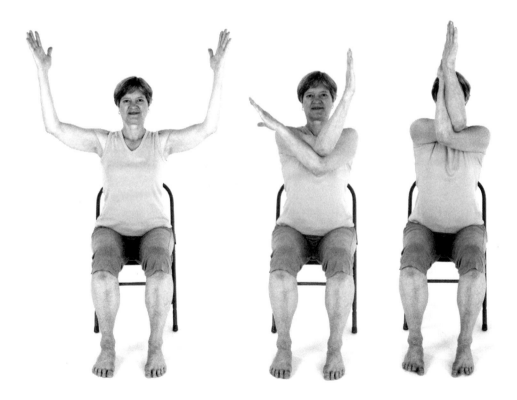

4. Hook your right elbow inside your left elbow crease.
5. Intertwine your forearms so that the fingers of your left hand hook onto the palm of your right hand.
6. Inhaling, lift from inside your chest and pull your upper arms back into the shoulder sockets.
7. Lift your elbows up, keeping your hands pointing straight up.
8. Remain like this for several breaths, then release and do the other side.

7. *CHAIR TWIST— See page 75.

8. *STANDING LUNGE WITH CHAIR— See page 72.

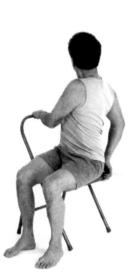

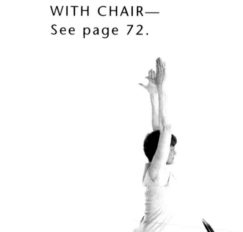

Using the chair for this twist will help to isolate the action in the spine, rotating every vertebra.

This standing pose develops hip flexibility, leg strength, and balance.

9. STANDING CRESCENT

Purpose: To mildly flex the lateral spine and to increase shoulder mobility.

Contraindications: Vertebral fracture, rotator cuff or impingement syndromes.

Prop: A wall.

Avoiding pitfalls: Keep your body carefully aligned with the side toward the wall. Avoid turning.

INSTRUCTIONS:

1. Stand with your left side a few inches from a wall. Lift your left arm high on the wall.
2. Test whether you are more comfortable with your palm or the back of your hand on the wall.
3. Firm your arm muscle; retain the upper arm deep within the shoulder joint.
4. Inhale, lift up through your torso, and lean sideways toward the wall until your hip and possibly your shoulder area touch the wall.
5. Lengthen your sides.
6. Gradually intensify this side stretch during several breaths.
7. You can step a little farther from the wall for a deeper stretch.
8. Repeat this movement several times; then turn and repeat on the other side.

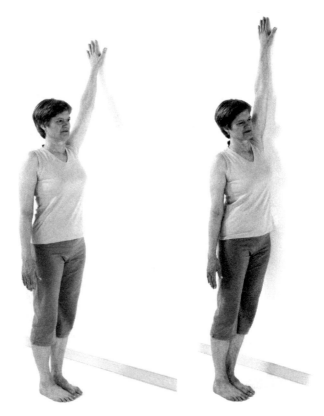

10. *ADHO MUKHA SVANASANA (Stage II, Wall Dog)—See Page 63.

11. *UTTHITA PARSVAKONASANA— See page 67.

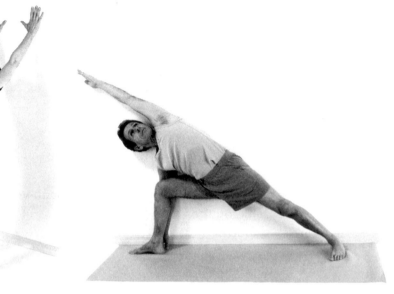

This pose provides a good neutralizing symmetrical spine and torso stretch.

This pose is an excellent hip opener, leg strengthener, and a gentle spinal twist.

12. *PRASARITA PADOTTANASANA—See page 71.

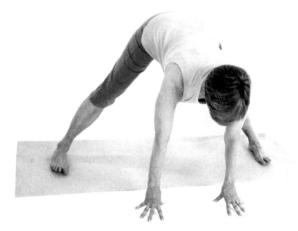

Avoid any spinal flexion in this pose.

Ankylosing Spondylitis *Asana*: Types of Motion

Name	Hip	Spine	Shoulder
■ **FUSED SPINE**			
Arms Clasped Behind	Extension	Mild extension	Extension
Strap Hanger			Abduction, external rotation
*Wall Dog	Flexion	Mild extension	Flexion, external rotation
Frog	Flexion, abduction, external rotation	Mild extension	External rotation, strength
Prasarita Padottanasana with Table	Flexion	Mild extension	Flexion
Garudasana Arms Only			Adduction, external rotation
Gomukhasana Arms Only			Flexion/extension, external rotation/internal rotation
Sitting Lunge with Chair	Flexion, extension	Mild extension	
*Windshield Wiper	Internal rotation, adduction	Mild rotation	Flexion, abduction
*Supta Padangusthasana	Flexion		Mild flexion
■ **UNFUSED SPINE**			
*Windshield Wiper	Adduction, internal rotation	Mild rotation	Flexion, abduction
*Bhujangasana	Extension	Extension	
Salabhasana	Extension	Extension	Extension, retraction
*Child's Pose	Flexion	Flexion/extension	Flexion
Gomukhasana	Flexion, adduction, external rotation		Flexion/extension, external rotation/internal rotation
Garudasana Arms Only			Adduction, external rotation
*Chair Twist	Flexion, adduction, abduction	Rotation	Retraction
*Standing Lunge with Chair	Flexion, extension	Mild extension	Retraction, depression
Standing Crescent	Adduction	Lateral flexion	Abduction, internal rotation
*Wall Dog	Flexion	Extension	Flexion, external rotation
*Utthita Parsvakonasana	Flexion, abduction, external rotation	Strengthen, rotate	Abduction, retraction, depression, elevation
*Prasarita Padottanasana	Flexion	Flexion	Retraction, depression

APPENDIX I

Alphabetical Index of Poses

Poses by Chapter

The All-Stars

these poses are preceded by an asterisk
when they are listed in other chapters

1. Tadasana, with variations: Tadasana Urdhva Hastasana, Tadasana Urdhva Baddha Hastasana
2. Standing Lunge with Wall
3. Adho Mukha Svanasana with four stages: Puppy, Wall Dog, Table Dog, Full Downward Dog
4. Utthita Parsvakonasana
5. Utthita Trikonasana
6. Prasarita Padottanasana
7. Standing Lunge with Chair
8. Pressure Cooker
9. Chair Twist
10. Wall Quad
11. Lotus Prep with Wall
12. Windshield Wiper
13. Setu Bandhasana
14. Supta Padangusthasana
15. Jathara Parivartanasana
16. Plank Series with three stages: Forearms and Knees, Forearms and Toes, Hands and Toes
17. Bhujangasana
18. Janu Sirsasana
19. Child's Pose
20. Savasana

The Shoulders

1. Wall Push-ups
2. Self-Hug with Belt
3. Parachute Pull
4. Stop
5. Arms Clasped Behind
6. Crossover Cactus
7. Gomukhasana Arms Only
8. Purvottanasana with Chair
9. *Adho Mukha Svanasana
10. *Plank Series
11. Vasisthasana Variation
12. *Jathara Parivartanasana
13. *Setu Bandhasana

The Hips

1. Corpse Roll
2. *Windshield Wiper
3. *Setu Bandhasana
4. *Supta Padangusthasana (with variation: One Knee to Chest)
5. *Lotus Prep with Wall
6. Baddha Konasana
7. *Janu Sirsasana
8. *Pressure Cooker
9. Eka Pada Supta Virasana
10. *Standing Lunge with Chair
11. Sitting Lunge with Chair
12. Gomukhasana Legs Only
13. *Utthita Parsvakonasana
14. *Utthita Trikonasana
15. *Prasarita Padottanasana

The Lumbar Spine

BEGINNING

1. *Windshield Wiper
2. Cat-Cow
3. Side Child's Pose
4. *Child's Pose
5. *Plank, Stage III

6. *Bhujangasana
7. Salabhasana
8. *Adho Mukha Svanasana, Stage II: Wall Dog
9. *Standing Lunge with Wall
10. Standing Crescent
11. *Pressure Cooker
12. *Chair Twist
13. Chair Malasana
14. *Setu Bandhasana
15. *Supta Padangusthasana

INTERMEDIATE

1. *Standing Lunge with Chair
2. *Utthita Trikonasana
3. *Utthita Parsvakonasana
4. Parivrtta Parsvakonasana
5. Uttanasana
6. Ardha Bhekasana
7. Ustrasana with Chair
8. Parighasana with Chair
9. Pigeon Pose with Bolster and Chair
10. *Janu Sirsasana
11. *Child's Pose

CHALLENGING

1. Viparita Dandasana Prep
2. Supta Virasana
3. Parivrtta Janu Sirsasana
4. Bharadvajasana
5. Ardha Matsyendrasana
6. Triang Mukhaikapada Paschimottanasana
7. Paschimottanasana

The Cervical Spine

1. *Tadasana
2. Cosmic Head Rest
3. The Thinker
4. *Chair Twist
5. Chair Malasana
6. Shoulders Back Head Forward
7. "Acha"

8. *Prasarita Padottanasana with Bent Knees
9. Slow Metronome
10. *Bhujangasana
11. *Jathara Parivartanasana
12. *Setu Bandhasana
13. Mountain Brook

The Knees

1. Chair Heel Slide
2. *Pressure Cooker
3. *Standing Lunge with Chair
4. *Lotus Prep with Wall
5. *Setu Bandhasana
6. *Supta Padangusthasana
7. *Janu Sirsasana
8. *Wall Quad
9. *Adho Mukha Svanasana
10. Utkatasana
11. *Utthita Parsvakonasana
12. Uttanasana

The Sacroiliac Joints

1. Tadasana with Block
2. *Windshield Wiper
3. *Lotus Prep with Wall
4. *Supta Padangusthasana
5. Bhujangasana (variation with shin belt)
6. Sukhasana
7. *Pressure Cooker
8. *Chair Twist
9. Chair Garudasana
10. *Standing Lunge with Chair
11. Standing Marichyasana III
12. Utthita Parsvakonasana (variation with chair)
13. Leaning Peacock
14. *Adho Mukha Svanasana, Stage II: Wall Dog
15. *Setu Bandhasana
16. Gomukhasana Legs Only
17. *Janu Sirsasana
18. Marichyasana I
19. *Jathara Parivartanasana
20. Pigeon Pose

21. *Child's Pose
22. *Savasana

The Wrists and Hands

1. Digital Roly Poly
2. Finger Push-ups
3. Anjali Mudra Series
4. Unseen Staff
5. Eka Digital Flexion
6. Stop
7. Eka Digital Extension
8. Aikido Wrist Stretches: Supinate and Twist, Pronate and Twist
9. Wall Finger Stretch
10. Parsvottanasana Prep
11. *Tadasana Urdhva Baddha Hastasana

The Feet and Ankles

1. *Tadasana
2. *Standing Lunge with Wall
3. *Supta Padangusthasana
4. *Lotus Prep with Wall
5. Utkatasana
6. Uttanasana with Rolled Blanket
7. *Utthita Parsvakonasana
8. *Utthita Trikonasana
9. *Prasarita Padottanasana
10. *Adho Mukha Svanasana
11. *Wall Quad
12. Virasana
13. Mulabandhasana (with two stages: One Foot, Both Feet)
14. Toe Abduction
15. Legs up the Wall

Scoliosis

GETTING TO KNOW YOUR CURVE

1. Tadasana with Side Bend
2. Side Child Spine
3. Exploratory Prasarita Padottanasana
4. Wall Dog/Table Dog

STRENGTHENING THE CONVEX SIDE

1. Seated Crescent Leveler
2. Resisted Abduction of Arm
3. Vasisthasana with four stages
4. Anantasana with two stages
5. Ardha Salabhasana Variation
6. Jathara Parivartanasana (variation with chair)

Ankylosing Spondylitis

FUSED SPINE

1. Arms Clasped Behind
2. Strap Hanger
3. *Adho Mukha Svanasana, Stage II: Wall Dog
4. Frog
5. Prasarita Padottanasana with Table
6. Garudasana Arms Only
7. Gomukhasana Arms
8. Sitting Lunge with Chair
9. *Windshield Wiper
10. *Supta Padangusthasana

UNFUSED SPINE

1. *Windshield Wiper
2. *Bhujangasana
3. Salabhasana
4. *Child's Pose
5. Gomukhasana
6. Garudasana Arms Only
7. *Chair Twist
8. *Standing Lunge with Chair
9. Standing Crescent
10. *Adho Mukha Svanasana, Stage II: Wall Dog
11. *Utthita Parsvakonasana
12. *Prasarita Padottanasana

Alignment Principles from Anusara Yoga

The yoga in this book derives from two main sources: B. K. S. Iyengar and John Friend. B. K. S. Iyengar's books are available for further study. John Friend is currently writing a definitive text of his work. In the meantime we offer a summary of the most relevant parts of his teaching, authorized by him.

The Alignment Principles from Anusara Yoga are designed to enhance the effectiveness of yoga practice, to make it much more subtle and powerful than simply holding a position of stretch. Every principle applies to every pose, and with time and practice, you can integrate them seamlessly and skillfully into your practice. The principles encompass three foundational elements: attitude (our intention and feeling), alignment (the precise placement of the body), and action (balancing strength and flexibility). There are correspondences between the principles, some being synergistic and others complementary to each other. They are included in the pose instructions in this book and are listed here as a summary.

Open to Grace: Begin the practice by pausing to soften, to become sensitive, and to recognize a bigger perspective that links your individual self to the universal. Become receptive to all possibilities in yourself and in the practice.

Foundation: The Foundation of any pose is the part that is on the floor or the seat of a chair. In the poses listed here it could be the feet, the hands, or the pelvic sitting bones. Root down evenly through all parts of the Foundation for stability. In the case of the hands and feet, the Foundation has four corners. See the illustration on page 235.

Inner Body Bright: Allow yourself to softly expand from deep inside. Feel your breath and deepen it, allowing your natural radiance to shine out. This is both a physical action and a subtle energetic opening.

Focal Point: A location in the body into which Muscular Energy collects to create stability, and out of which one expands with Organic Energy. There are three Focal Points, as illustrated on page 311, and only the one that is most weight bearing and closest to the Foundation is active in any given pose. When you are standing or sitting, the pelvis Focal Point is active. When the weight is on the hands, such as in Adho Mukha Svanasana, the heart Focal Point is active. The palate Focal Point is used for inverted poses such as headstand and shoulder stand, which are not described in this book.

Muscular Energy: The muscles contract and support the bones from all sides, and connect the limbs into the midline and into the torso, providing stability and strength. The main current of muscular flow is from the periphery of the body toward the Focal Point of the pose.

Inner Spiral: This action is an expanding spiral that begins at the feet and moves up the legs to the top of the pelvis. Its three primary effects are (1) the thighs turn inward, move back, and then spread apart, widening the pelvis; (2) the lower back arches; and (3) the groins soften.

Outer Spiral: This spiral begins at the top of the pelvis and moves down around each leg, narrowing as it goes, and ending at the outer edge of the heel. The tailbone lengthens down, the buttocks firm without squeezing too tightly, and the legs turn out just enough to balance the inward turning of Inner Spiral. The Outer Spiral provides stability and groundedness.

Organic Energy: From the Focal Point of the pose, extend energetically down into the Foundation, up through the top of your head, and out through your arms. This principle helps to make the poses more fluid and expansive.

Shins-In-Thighs-Out: This action of pulling the shins toward the midline and the thighs away from the midline will improve the alignment of the knees and also benefit the lower back.

The Loops: The Loops are refined actions that align the designated segments of the body in relation to each other in the vertical plumb-line. The Loops help to create equal support and freedom in the front and back of the body. There are seven pairs of Loops, each pair having one on the right and one on the left at each level. Each Loop has a particular direction of flow (either up the front and down the back, or vice versa) and they interlock like gears at the intersection points (see accompanying diagram). Some Loops have more of a feeling of strength and stabilization (the Ankle, Shin, Thigh, Pelvis, and Shoulder Loops) and others have more of a feeling of lift away from the pull of gravity (Kidney and Skull Loops). A student might activate one Loop more on one side than another when addressing bodily asymmetries. Some poses may require extra focus on a certain Loop, which is noted in the instructions.

Some of the beneficial effects of the Loops include the following: The **Ankle Loop** roots the back of the heels down and lifts the inner arches up, stabi-

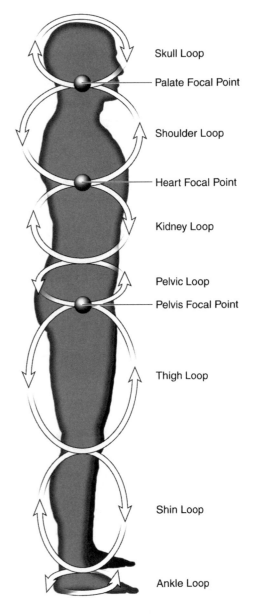

Figure 21. *The three Focal Points and the location and direction of the seven Loops.*

lizing the stance. The **Shin Loop** activates the calf muscles and keeps the tops of the shins from moving back too far as they do in hyperextension of the knees. The **Thigh Loop** lifts up the quadriceps muscles and moves the tops of the thighs back, which is beneficial for the hips and lower back. The **Pelvic Loop** moves the tailbone and pelvic bones down, lengthening the lower back, and also lifts the abdomen up. The **Kidney Loop** lifts and softens the back of the ribs, lifting the weight of the chest off the lumbar spine. It also softens the front of the chest. The **Shoulder Loop** tilts the head slightly back, maintaining the cervical curvature. It moves down the back of the neck and shoulder blades. At the lower tips of the shoulder blades it moves forward and lifts the front of the chest up. This loop provides essential support for the arms and head. The **Skull Loop** moves the base of the skull back and up, lightens the head on the neck, and softens the eyes.

Balanced Action: The principles all reflect the balance of opposite currents of energy and action in the body (in and out, up and down, etc.). This balance brings a dynamic stability so that the poses are not rigid, collapsed, or mechanical, but alive, well organized, and expressive.

Glossary

abduction Movement away from the midline. Lifting one's arms to either side abducts them.

abductor hallucis A muscle that brings the great toe away from the other toes, originating at the calcaneus and the soft tissues nearby, and inserting at the outside of the proximal bone of the great toe.

acetabulum The large spherical indentation in the pelvic bone that forms the pelvic side of the hip joint.

Achilles bursitis See *bursitis*.

Achilles tendonitis Inflammation of the Achilles tendon, generally occurring just above the heel bone, into which the tendon inserts, attaching the gastrocnemius and soleus muscles to the calcaneus.

acromioclavicular joint The joint connecting the clavicle with the acromion, a superolateral boney projection of the scapula.

acromion A boney projection of the scapula, or shoulder blade, that joins it to the lateral clavicle, or collarbone.

adduction Movement toward the midline, even crossing it. To touch one's left shoulder with the right hand, one must adduct the right arm.

ankle mortise The space between the distal ends of the tibia and fibula into which the uppermost bone of the foot, the talus, just fits.

ankylosing spondylitis Hereditary progressive inflammation and eventual fusion of vertebral bodies, largely in males. Fusion and virtual rigidity of the spine are frequently complete by the early twenties, yielding a stooped or hunched thorax.

anterior In the front.

Anusara Yoga principles of alignment See Appendix III.

arterial insufficiency A condition chiefly affecting older individuals in which the vascular system is unable to transport enough blood to supply adequate oxygen and nutrients to the periphery, including the muscles.

arthritis Destructive inflammation of a joint or joints. When one is referring to types of arthritis, the plural is *arthritides*, in the manner of ancient Greek.

asana Sanskrit term for yoga pose or poses, literally translated as "seat" or "posture." The term is both singular and plural.

axon The thin extended outgrowth from a neuron that normally propagates impulses away from that neuron toward another neuron, a muscle, or a gland. The term derives from the Greek word for "axis."

brachial plexus The complex rearrangement of cervical nerve roots after they leave the cervical spine, taking place in the lateral neck and upper inner chest area. In the course of this reorganization, the nerve fibers form trunks, divisions, and cords—all part of the plexus—which subsequently become the major nerves to the upper extremities (e.g., the median, ulnar, and radial nerves).

bridging spondylitis An arthritic condition in which two or more vertebrae are either fused together or have dangerously large osteophytes, in either case severely limiting range of motion at that joint. Usually this occurs in the cervical spine of older people, where it may or may not be associated with HLA-B27 as a very mild form of ankylosing spondylitis; it need not be genetic.

bursa A closed sac with synovial lining and joint fluid within, generally separating a bone from a tendon. The bursae are thought to have evolved from joints, since they have the same basic structure, and to have been retained because they prevent the tendon from bruising the bone, and the bone from fraying the tendon. The Latin word *bursa* means "purse."

bursitis Inflammation of a bursa (see above), which can become quite painful. Examples are Achilles bursitis (between the tendon and the ankle bone), prepatellar bursitis (external to the kneecap), pes anserinus bursitis (separating the sartorius, gracilis, and semitendinosus tendons from the tibia just below the inner knee), and ischial bursitis (between the bones on which one sits and the hamstring muscles that attach to them).

carpal tunnel syndrome Entrapment of the median nerve in a tight-fitting passageway between the bones of the wrist. Tendons also pass through the carpal tunnel and injure the nerve when they become inflamed or swollen (e.g., when swelling in pregnancy congests the compartment). This syndrome causes pain and numbness of the palmar side of the thumb, index, and middle fingers, and the thumb side of the ring finger, and weakness in lifting the thumb perpendicular to the plane of the palm.

cartilage The semi-stiff substance that lines joints and forms movable tubes in the body such as the trachea, the nasal cavity, and the Adam's apple. There are three forms: hyaline cartilage, elastic cartilage, and fibrocartilage.

cauda equina Collections of nerve fibers, rootlets, that descend through the lumbar portion of the canal, giving the appearance of a horse's tail, hence, the name *cauda equina*. In adults, the spinal cord proper ends at the lower thoracic levels, far above where lumbar nerve roots exit the spinal canal.

cerebrovascular disease Blood vessel abnormalities in the brain, including aneurysm, stroke, intracranial hemorrhage, and changes in small blood vessels of the brain caused by hypertension.

cervical spine The seven vertebrae of the neck.

cervical vertebral instability When, because of fracture or serious disruption, the cervical vertebral column is vulnerable to gross malalignment, exposing the spinal column within to sudden catastrophic injury.

Chiari malformations A range of congenital defects at the base of the skull that might be mild, with dizziness, neuromuscular symptoms, and impaired coordination (type I); might involve defects of the cervical vertebrae and spinal canal, which might lead to paralysis (type II, Arnold-Chiari); or might even be more serious, causing hydrocephalus and similar difficulties (type III).

chondrocytes Cells that secrete the fibers that constitute cartilage.

chondromalacia patellae Softening of the cartilage of the kneecap. Because the knee is an elliptical joint involving three bones, the back of the kneecap is cut with fine facets, almost like a precious jewel, so that it fits properly over the joint between the tibia and the femur at all angles. Malalignment in the knee, which then contributes to degenerative changes in the cartilage, can cause pain. Also known as *runner's knee*, it is more common in women, with onset usually before age forty.

coccygodynia Pain in the region of the coccyx, frequently due to a fracture or dislocation at the sacrococcygeal junction, itself often the result of trauma such as a fall.

collagen A component of connective tissue that is pervasive throughout the body. It is a triple helix of three long protein chains that wrap around one another. Cross-linked molecules of collagen greatly resist stretch and are stronger than many metals.

collateral ligaments, medial and lateral Tough cartilaginous thongs that attach the tibia and fibula to the femur at the inner and outer areas of the knee. The most common pathology of these ligaments is sprain. They can also be stretched, giving the knee "wiggle room" and leading to valgum and varus deformities. In addition, they can tear along with the menisci.

contralateral The opposite side (e.g., the right is contralateral to the left).

conus medullaris The enlargement of the spinal cord at the lowest thoracic level, where it gives rise to the fibers for all five lumbar levels that make up the cauda equina. The conus medullaris is where the spinal cord proper terminates.

cruciate ligaments, anterior and posterior Strong cords of fibrous tissue that restrain the tibia from moving forward and backward, respectively, at the knee.

de Quervain's syndrome Inflammation (tenosynovitis) of the tendons of the thumb muscles—the abductor pollicis longus, extensor pollicis brevis, and extensor pollicis longus—at the radial bone's styloid process (dorsal wrist).

dendrite The branching outgrowth from a neuron that acquires impulses, which are then transmitted through the cell body to the axon and, hence, to another cell. The Greek word for *dendrites* means "pertaining to a tree."

distal Farther from the point of reference or axis (e.g., the hand is distal to the elbow).

Dupuytren's contracture Hereditary shortening and thickening of the flexor tendons of the hand, generally beginning after middle age with the fourth digit and sometimes progressing to involve several.

effusion Collection of fluid beyond what is physiologically required. This can occur in joints, distorting the relationships and movement patterns of the bones, or in other places (e.g., pulmonary effusion).

elastin A component of connective tissue made up of polypeptide (protein) chains that cross-link like collagen but with the opposite effect: they coil into a form that may uncoil when the fiber is stretched, and resile (recoil) when the stretch is terminated.

eversion Lateral movement of the foot toward the little toe side and a lifting up of that side, producing an outward-facing sole.

extension Motion of bones at a joint away from each other or away from the torso. Exception: Ankle and toe extension bring the foot and toes upward.

facet syndrome Painful spinal condition resulting from arthritis or other mechanical problems in the facet joints of the vertebrae. There are no neurological sequelae such as paresthesias, numbness, weakness, or sciatica. Recent literature suggests that many cases identified as facet syndrome are actually segmental rigidity, simple tightening of the longitudinal muscles along the spine.

external rotation Clockwise revolving motion of the right arm and leg; counterclockwise revolving of the left limbs. At the ankle and wrist, these movements are termed *supination*.

fibrocartilaginous triangle Tough diagonal tendinous bands that essentially hold the skeleton of the hand together from the palm side.

flexion Motion of bones toward one another at a joint generally to the functional position, toward the front. One exception is ankle and toe flexion, which to physicians means pointing the foot and toes downward.

gait cycle The repetitive series of movements that each foot, ankle, knee, and hip and the trunk and arms go through with each pair of steps.

gastroesophageal reflux Nonphysiological flow of digestive juices and eaten material back to the esophagus from the stomach. This can be due to weak gastroesophageal sphincter muscles, but rarely occurs after inverted yoga poses unless it also occurs when the practitioner is right-side up. Those with GERD (gastroesophageal reflux disease) should not do yoga for five hours after eating.

genu valgum Inward tilting of the knee joint, toward the other knee.

genu varus Outward tilting of the knee joint, away from the other knee.

glenoid fossa The shallow cup-shaped part of the scapula into which the humerus (upper arm bone) fits to form the shoulder joint.

golfer's elbow Inflammation of the inside (medial side) of the elbow, generally involving the tendons of the muscles that flex the wrist, or the connective tissue to which they are attached.

Golgi tendon organs Sensory nerve endings embedded in each tendon's fibers that send signals inhibiting the contraction of the muscle to which the tendon is attached. The Golgi tendon organs are stimulated by passive stretch or active contraction of the muscle—anything that stretches the tendon. Their inhibitory output is proportional to the stretch and does not change regardless of how long the muscle remains stretched. They are named after their discoverer, Nobel laureate Camillo Golgi (1843–1926).

gout Generally intermittent, extremely painful condition deriving from the body's overproduction of uric acid, a derivative of the nucleic acid purine. It is associated with a protein-rich diet and related to obesity.

herniated nucleus pulposus Rupture of a protruding nucleus pulposus, the soft inner mass (jello-like) of an intervertebral disc, through the annulus fibrosus, the relatively stiff outer (rice paper–like) membrane of the disc. Unfortunately these herniations almost invariably occur in a posterior direction, where the neurological material within the spine is located.

Hill-Sachs deformity Fracture of the medial humeral head, usually requiring special posterior oblique X-rays or MRI to detect.

humerus The bone of the upper arm.

hyperlordosis Abnormal arching of the spine with convexity forward. It is found most commonly in the lumbar spine, but can occur in the cervical and even (rarely) the thoracic spine.

idiopathic Without cause.

iliopsoas Primary hip flexing muscles originating at the lateral edges of the lumbar vertebrae (*psoas*) and the inner surface of the pelvis (*iliacus*) and attaching to the inner upper region of the femurs.

impingement syndrome Where movement or positioning causes compression, usually of a tendon. In shoulder impingement, the supraspinatus tendon is pressed between the acromion and the head of the humerus.

inferior Below.

inguinal hernia Often painful protrusion of the abdominal cavity linings, and possibly some intestine, through the abdominal wall at the groin. This hernia is more common in men. There is usually an abdominal bulge that resolves with lying down. Bulges that do not resolve may become lodged between the abdominal wall and the deeper muscles and skin, a dangerous condition, known as *incarceration*, demanding immediate medical attention.

internal rotation Counterclockwise revolving motion of the right arm and leg; clockwise revolving of the left limbs. At the ankle and wrist, these movements are termed *pronation*.

intertriginous dermatitis Skin condition located in the skin between the digits.

intrafusal fibers Sensory nerve endings embedded in tiny muscle fibers, themselves embedded in every skeletal muscle. When stretched, the intrafusal fibers send facilitatory signals affecting the large muscle in which they are embedded, stimulating that particular muscle to contract more strongly. The tiny muscles adjust the sensitivity of the intrafusal fibers to stretch, damping down their facilitatory signal output if a muscle is stretched for any length of time. They are responsible for the stretch, or myotatic, reflex.

intrinsic muscles Muscles of the hands and feet that are located entirely in the hands and feet themselves. In contrast, most muscles that move the extremities, especially those used for more powerful actions, are located in the forearms and lower legs, with long tendons to the fingers and toes. Any other arrangement would be too bulky and produce too much momentum in the hands and feet for the deft movements required of the extremities.

inversion Movement of the foot in which the inner arch lifts up and the foot turns in toward the midline.

ischial bursitis See *bursitis.*

labral tear Injury to the fibrocartilaginous ring around most major joints. The shoulder joint, for example, has posterior, anterior, superior, and lateral labra. The superior labrum is often damaged in an anterior-posterior direction (SLAP lesion). In the hip, labral tears are common in dancers and yoga students. However, the anterior joint capsular fibers are very strong and resist tearing, as they counterbalance the trunk's weight during walking. Labral tears are painful, and difficult to diagnose without MRI.

lateral Toward the side.

latissimus dorsi Large muscles connecting the back of the pelvis to the inner upper area of the humerus. Their primary action is to rotate and bring the arms inward and behind the body.

ligamentum flavum A yellowish ligament that extends the entire length of the spine, lining the rear portion of the long spinal canal that the nerves pass through on their way from the brain to the arms and legs and body.

longitudinal arch The rising curve of the inner foot that distributes weight to the heel and ball of the foot. Its keystone is the navicular bone.

lordosis The normal convexity-forward arching of the lumbar and cervical spine.

lumbar spine The five vertebrae at the lower end of the spine, from the level of the twelfth rib to the sacrum.

macular degeneration Loss of cellular function in the most sensitive part of the eye. In the wet form of macular degeneration, new blood vessel formation crowds out some of the light-sensitive cells. Their rupture and subsequent hemorrhage damages the macula, potentially causing vision to deteriorate substantially. In the more common dry form, pigmented areas (drusen) impair vision much less.

medial Toward the midline.

meniscus, medial and lateral The cartilage inside the knee joint that improves the fit between the tibia and the femur and cushions both during weight bearing.

myotatic reflex Contraction of a muscle in response to a sudden stretching force, due to stretch of the intrafusal fibers (e.g., the patellar reflex, the Achilles tendon reflex).

neck of the femur The diagonal part at the upper end of the femur, from the greater trochanter at the side to the rounded head in the actual hip socket. This buttress shape allows for greater stability in walking than we would have if the femur were one long straight bone. Wolff's law describes how the sideward forces generated during walking gradually remodel the femur to have a diagonal neck. Babies are born without that angle at the greater trochanter.

neuroforamen Space through which a nerve root passes that is created by the fit of two adjoining vertebrae. Plural: neuroforamina.

Neutral The position of limbs or torso that is without flexion, extension, abduction, adduction, or external or internal rotation. The entire body in neutral is also known as the "anatomical position." This is different from the yogi's Savasana, in which arms and legs are somewhat externally rotated.

nonsteroidal anti-inflammatory drugs Medications related to aspirin which interfere with the prostaglandin-mediated pathways that generate pain and enhance inflammation. These medicines reduce both pain and inflammatory responses, such as swelling and redness. However, their use is associated with varying degrees of side effects, such as gastric irritation, ulcer, and prolonged bleeding time. Examples are Motrin, Relafen, Voltaren, Celebrex, and Mobic.

nutation Movement of the sacrum in any plane. Some researchers give evidence that the sacrum actually moves around diagonal axes (i.e., from lower right to upper left or lower left to upper right).

osteoarthritis Erosion of the cartilage at joints, either without single cause or due to trauma. It is characterized by irregular boney outgrowths at the joint, and painful restrictions of movement and swelling mainly of weight-bearing and very active joints. Since chronic conditions are cumulative, it is more common in older persons.

osteoarthropathy Any disorder that affects bones and joints. Its origins are Greek: *osteo* (bone) + *arthron* (joint) + *pathos* (suffering).

osteoblasts Cells that line the outside of bones and are destined to make the protein matrix of the bones.

osteocytes Cells descended from osteoblasts, located within the bones, that actively secrete the protein matrix and are surrounded by it.

osteophytes Irregular nonanatomical boney growths at or near joints, associated with osteoarthritis. They may limit range of motion of the joints and in the spine. Since the facet joints are so near the neuroforamina, they can also painfully compress the nerve roots as they exit the spinal canal. Greek: *osteo* (bone) + *phyton* (plant).

osteoporosis Reduction of bone mineral, and thereby bone strength beyond 2.5 standard deviations of the mean, which is equivalent to bones weaker than 99 percent of healthy thirty-year-old women.

paraspinal muscles Near-midline longitudinal muscles that attach to and move the vertebrae.

paresthesias Strange sensations such as tingling, of being stuck by pins and needles, or of insects crawling on the skin. *Numbness* is when you do not feel what is there; paresthesias are when you feel what is not there.

patellofemoral arthralgia Pain brought about by improper fitting of the underside of the kneecap, or patella, and the forward face of the femoral condyles at the knee joint.

pectoralis major and minor Muscles connecting the scapula and upper humerus to the ribs and sternum.

perichondrium Lining such as that between the ends of bones and the cartilage that supplies oxygen and nourishes the chondrocytes, cells that make cartilage.

plantar fascia The tough membrane that connects the heel to the toes. Like a bowstring, the plantar fascia puts the foot under tension that bends the middle of its underside upward, maintaining the longitudinal arch of the foot.

plantar fasciitis Painful inflammation of the insertion of the plantar fascia into the calcaneus, also known as "heel spur."

pontine Related to the pons, part of the brain that integrates motor and sensory signals between the spinal cord and higher brain regions such as the cerebral cortex.

posterior In the rear.

prepatellar bursitis See *bursitis.*

protraction Movement of the scapulae (shoulder blades) forward, toward the ventral, or navel-bearing side of the body. In human anatomy, it is nearly equivalent to abducting them, that is, bringing them away from the spine.

proximal Closer to the point of reference or axis.

pseudogout Goutlike episodes caused by calcium pyrophosphate crystals, rather than the urate crystals that irritate the synovial membrane in true gout. It is also associated with calcification of the articular cartilage, known as *chondrocalcinosis.*

quadriceps The prominent muscle at the front of the thigh that straightens the knee.

radiculopathy Compression or injury to the nerve roots that exit the spine.

Reiter's syndrome Autoimmune arthritis following a bacterial infection of the intestines or genitourinary system, generally affecting joints of the lower extremities and the ligaments and tendons that cross them. Also known as *reactive arthritis*, it may be accompanied by palmar or plantar rash, oral or genital sores, and inflammation of the eyes.

retraction Movement of the scapulae (shoulder blades) backward, toward the dorsal aspect of the thorax. In human anatomy, it is nearly equivalent to adducting them, that is, bringing them toward the spine.

retrolisthesis See *spondylolisthesis.*

rheumatoid arthritis Arthritic damage to joints resulting from the immune system's actions, generally on the joint capsules' lining or synovium.

rotator cuff syndrome or tear The rotator cuff consists of the supraspinatus, infraspinatus, teres minor, and subscapularis muscles, which secure the humerus into the shoulder socket. A rip in the fabric of any of these technically qualifies as rotator cuff syndrome. Usually rotator cuff syndrome includes the supraspinatus tendon, whether other muscles or tendons are involved or not. Supraspinatus tears cause pain when lifting the arm between 80 and 120 degrees.

sacroiliac joint A bilateral synovial joint between the outer edges of the sacrum and the inner edges of the iliac bones.

sacroiliitis Inflammation of the sacroiliac joint.

sacrum Spade-shaped central posterior pelvic bone that articulates with the iliac bones on either side (the sacroiliac joints), with the lowest lumbar vertebra above (L5-S1 joint), and with the coccyx below.

scapulothoracic The large area between the shoulder blade, or scapula, and the backs of ribs 2 through 6, over which the shoulder blade normally moves. It is often referred to as a joint, although its size and structure are quite different from any other joint.

scoliosis Lateral curvature of the spine, often with a rotation as well. The curve is described by its location, as in "left thoracolumbar scoliosis." Idiopathic scoliosis disappears with forward bending.

sesamoid bone A bone encapsulated within a tendon and named for its shape, which resembles a sesame seed. There is one in the flexor tendon of the big toe as it rounds the joint that connects the toe to the foot. The patella is the largest sesamoid bone in the human body.

SLAP lesion Tear of the superior labrum of the shoulder joint, occurring in an anterior-posterior direction where the long head of the biceps tendon crosses just above the joint.

spinal cord The part of the central nervous system that descends within the vertebral column, conducting nearly all motor and sensory communications between the body and the brain. The cord is divided into cervical (neck), thoracic (where the ribs are), and lumbar (from the ribs to the pelvis) regions.

spinal stenosis Narrowing of the inside of the central canal of the spine, which is formed by the column of vertebrae. This canal houses the spinal cord (see above). The narrowing can be due to an intervertebral disc that bulges or has herniated at a specific level; a thickening of the bones, which can narrow whole sections of the spinal canal; or a swollen ligamentum flavum, which can narrow variable stretches of the canal. The pain, numbness, weakness, and paresthesias that result from this type of compression of the nerve fibers are usually somewhat symmetrical.

spondyloarthropathy See *ankylosing spondylitis.*

spondylolisthesis The undesired sliding of one vertebra (generally forward) on the one below it. The displacement is graded (grade I = 1–25 percent, grade II = 25–50 percent, etc.). It can result in narrowing of the central canal (stenosis) or it may narrow a neuroforamen, causing radiculopathy. Displacement may also be posterior (retrolisthesis) or sideways (lateral listhesis).

spondylolysis Separation of the facet-bearing part of a vertebra from the vertebral body. This can occur by traumatic fracture of the pars intraarticularis and is believed to be congenital in some cases.

sprain Where at least some of the fibers of the ligaments that bind a joint together are torn apart. A *strain* is stretching without a tear.

stretch reflex The same as the myotatic reflex (see above).

superior Above.

suprascapular nerve entrapment Rupture of the ligament that holds the suprascapular nerve, which reaches from its origins at C5–C6 over the top of the scapula through the suprascapular notch to serve the supraspinatus and infraspinatus muscles, within the suprascapular notch, causing the nerve to slide back and forth or even leave the notch altogether, subjecting it to damage. This is sometimes seen in pitchers and back-bending yogis.

synapse The site where impulses are passed from one neuron to another, generally by neurotransmitter molecules but sometimes by direct (electronic) propagation of the signal. This communication involves a one-way, all-or-nothing excitation of the stimulated neuron, though recent observations question the all-or-nothing, the one-way, and other aspects of the Hodgkin-Huxley theory that lies at the foundation of most computational neurobiology. (For more on this, see B. Gutkin and G. B. Ermentrout, "Spikes too kinky in the cortex?" *Nature* 440 [April 20, 2006]: 999–1000.) The word originates from the Greek *syn* (together) and *hapto* (to clasp).

synovial fluid The yellowish white fluid that bathes each joint. This fluid serves three essential purposes: it is a first-class lubricant; it brings oxygen, food, and protein-building blocks to the cartilage of the joint; and it protects the joint from many mechanical and biological causes of disruption.

synovial membrane A membrane, similar to a gasket, that seals the synovial fluid in the joint. It is quite vascular and richly invested with nerves, secretes and resorbs the synovial fluid, and is exquisitely sensitive, causing pain with distention, inflammation, or disruption.

tennis elbow A small but painful tear in the forearm's extensor aponeurosis, a broad flat tendon on the dorsal forearm. It occurs when the muscles that lift the hand and fingers are stressed, as in backhand.

teres major and minor Small muscles attaching the outer scapula to the humerus, rotating it internally and externally, respectively.

thoracic outlet syndrome Entrapment of the brachial plexus, or the nerves that emerge from it, at the neck or upper chest (generally either between the scalenii, by an anomalous rib that is attached to a cervical vertebra, beneath the clavicle, or at the coracoid process). Except when the nerves are entrapped between two cervical muscles, blood vessels may be involved.

thoracic spine The twelve vertebrae at the level of the chest, between the neck and the lower back, to which the ribs attach.

vagus nerve A nerve that exits the brain through the skull and descends bilaterally through the neck and torso to influence the heart, lungs, and digestive system. This nerve is an exception to the rule that all communication between the body and the brain occurs by virtue of the spinal cord.

vasovagal episode Abrupt changes in abdominal or thoracic pressure (e.g., when voiding, or when in an airplane or headstand) that can trigger the vagus nerve to slow down the heart, at times causing fainting.

voluntary subluxation Repeated separation of the humerus from the glenoid fossa, a very painful form of shoulder joint abnormality that can happen without trauma in people prone to it. If it happens twice, corrective surgery is suggested.

zygapophyseal joints Referring to the facet joints that link each vertebra to the one above and the one below it. From the Greek root *zugon*, meaning "yoke," possibly because these joint surfaces are somewhat ovoid.

Notes

Author's Note

1. Jacob Burckhardt, *Weltgeschichtliche Betrachtungen*, 1905, p. 147, quoted in Johan Huizinga, *The Autumn of the Middle Ages*, translated by Rodney J. Payton and Ulrich Mammitzsch (Chicago: University of Chicago Press, 1996), p. 174.

2. Sam Harris, *The End of Faith: Religion, Terror and the Future of Reason* (New York: W. W. Norton, 2004), chap. 2.

Chapter 1

1. F. Berenbaum, *Osteoarthritis: Epidemiology, Pathology and Pathogenesis. Primer on the Rheumatic Diseases*, 12th ed. (Atlanta: Arthritis Foundation, 2001).

2. Centers for Disease Control, Behavioral Risk Factor Surveillance System, 2003.

3. L. Ala-Kokko, C. T. Baldwin, et al., "Single base mutation in the type II pro-*collagen* gene (COL2A1) as a cause of primary osteoarthritis associated with a mild chondrodysplasia," *Proceedings of the National Academy of Sciences of the United States of America* 87, no. 17 (1990): 6565–6568.

4. R. G. Knowlton, et al., "Genetic linkage of a polymorphism in the type II pro*collagen* gene (COL2A1) to primary osteoarthritis associated with a mild chondrodysplasia," *New England Journal of Medicine* 322, no. 8 (1990): 526–530.

5. M. Garfinkel, H. R. Schumacher, et al., "Effect of joint motion on experimental calcium pyrophosphate dehydrated crystal induced arthritis," *Journal of Rheumatology* 17 (1990): 644–655.

6. M. Garfinkel, H. R. Schumacher, et al., "Effect of joint motion on experi-

mental calcium pyrophosphate dehydrated crystal induced arthritis," *Journal of Rheumatology* 17 (1990): 644–655. M. Garfinkel, "Yoga as a complementary therapy," *Geriatrics Aging* 9, no. 3 (2006): 190–194. M. Garfinkel and H. R. Schumacher, "Yoga," *Rheumatic Diseases Clinics of North America* 26, no. 1 (February 2000): 125–132, x.

7. R. C. Lawrence, C. Helmick, et al., "Estimates of the prevalence of arthritis and selected musculoskeletal disorders in the United States," *Arthritis and Rheumatism* 41, no. 5 (1998): 778–789.

8. M. Renoux, P. Hilliquin, et al., "Cellular activation products in osteoarthritis synovial fluid," *International Journal of Clinical Pharmacology Research* 15, no. 4 (1995): 135–138.

9. R. C. Lawrence, C. Helmick, et al., "Estimates of the prevalence of arthritis and selected musculoskeletal disorders in the United States," *Arthritis and Rheumatism* 41, no. 5 (1998): 778–789.

10. R. Zenz, R. Eferl, et al., "Psoriasis-like skin disease and arthritis caused by inducible epidermal deletion of Jun proteins," *Nature* 437 (September 15, 2005): 369–375.

11. Ibid.

12. National Psoriasis Foundation Web site at www.psoriasis.org.

13. I. B. Lobov, S. Rao, et al., "WNT7b mediates macrophage-induced programmed cell death in patterning of the vasculature," *Nature* 437 (September 15, 2005): 417–421.

14. D. S. Pisetsky and S. F. Trien, *The Duke University Medical Center Book of Arthritis* (New York: Ballantine Books, 1991).

15. R. C. Lawrence, C. Helmick, et al., "Estimates of the prevalence of arthritis and selected musculoskeletal disorders in the United States," *Arthritis and Rheumatism* 41, no. 5 (1998): 778–789.

16. H. K. Choi, K. Atkinson, et al., "Purine-rich foods, dairy and protein intake, and the risk of gout in men," *New England Journal of Medicine* 350, no. 11 (2004): 1093–1103.

17. H. K. Choi, K. Atkinson, et al., "Obesity, weight change, hypertension, diuretic use, and risk of gout in men: The health professionals follow-up study," *Archives of Internal Medicine* 165, no. 7 (2005): 742–748.

18. Sp. Johnsen, H. Larsson, et al., "Risk of hospitalization for myocardial infarction among uses or rofecoxib, celecoxib and other NSAIDs: A population-based case-control study," *Archives of Internal Medicine* 165, no. 9 (2005): 978–984. J. Hippisley-Cox and C. Coupland, "Risk of myocardial infarction in patients taking cyclo-oxygenase-2 inhibitors or conventional

non-steroidal anti-inflammatory drugs: Population based case-control analysis," *BMJ* 330, no. 7504 (2005): 1366. P. Emery, A. Moore, and D. Hawkey, "Increased risk of cardiovascular events with coxibs and NSAIDs," *Lancet* 365, no. 9470 (2005): 1538.

19. D. J. Felson, Y. Zhang, et al., "Weight loss reduces the risk of symptomatic knee arthritis in women. The Framingham Study," *Annals of Internal Medicine* 116, no. 7 (1992): 598–599.

20. D. S. Pisetsky and S. F. Trien, *The Duke University Medical Center Book of Arthritis* (New York: Ballantine Books, 1991). M. A. Minor, J. E. Hewett, et al., "Efficacy of physical conditioning exercise in patients with rheumatoid arthritis or osteoarthritis," *Arthritis and Rheumatism* 32 (1989): 1397–1405. M. Munneke, et al., "Effect of a high-intensity weight-bearing exercise program on radiologic damage progression of the large joints in subgroups of patients with rheumatoid arthritis," *Arthritis and Rheumatism* 53, no. 3 (2005): 410–417. M. A. Melikoglu, S. Karatay, et al., "Association between dynamic exercise therapy and IGF-1 and IGFBP-3 concentrations in the patients with rheumatoid arthritis," *Rheumatology International* 4 (February 26, 2006): 309–313. L. Maxwell and P. Tugwell, "High-intensity exercise for rheumatoid arthritis was associated with less joint damage of the hands and feet than physical therapy," *American College of Physicians Journal Club* 142, no. 3 (2005): 73. C. H. Van Gool, B. W. Penninx, et al., "Effects of exercise adherence on physical function among overweight older adults with knee osteoarthritis," *Arthritis and Rheumatism* 53, no. 1 (2005): 24–32.

21. S. L. Kolasinski, M. Garfinkel, et al., "Iyengar yoga for treating symptoms of the knees: A pilot study," *Journal of Alternative and Complementary Medicine* 11, no. 4 (August 11, 2005): 689–693. M. Garfinkel and H. R. Schumacher Jr., "Yoga," *Rheumatic Diseases Clinics of North America* 26, no. 1 (February 2000): 125–132, x. M. S. Garfinkel, H. R. Schumacher Jr., et al., "Evaluation of a yoga based regimen for treatment of osteoarthritis of the hands," *Journal of Rheumatology* 21, no. 12 (December 1994): 2341–2343.

CHAPTER 2

1. Alistair Shearer (trans.), *The Yoga Sutra of Patanjali* (New York: Bell Tower, 1982), p. 24.

2. "Yoga in America," Harris Interactive Service Bureau, February 5, 2005, at www.yogajournal.com, accessed April 16, 2006.

3. Georg Feuerstein, *The Yoga Tradition* (Prescott, Ariz.: Hohm Press, 1998), pp. 80–85.

4. A. Cushman, "New Light on Yoga," *Yoga Journal* (July/August 1999): 44–49.

5. I. K. Taimni, *The Science of Yoga* (Wheaton, Ill.: Theosophical Publishing House, 1972), pp. 6–10.

6. L. Long, A. Huntley, and E. Ernst, "Which complementary and alternative therapies benefit which conditions? A survey of the opinions of 223 professional organizations," *Complementary Therapies in Medicine* 9, no. 3 (September 2001): 178–185.

7. B. S. Oken, S. Kishiyama, et al., "Randomized controlled trial of yoga and exercise in multiple sclerosis," *Neurology* 62, no. 11 (June 8, 2004): 2058–2064.

8. M. S. Garfinkel, H. R. Schumacher Jr., et al., "Evaluation of a yoga based regimen for treatment of osteoarthritis of the hands," *Journal of Rheumatology* 21, no. 12 (December 1994): 2341–2343. M. Garfinkel, "Yoga as a complementary therapy," *Geriatrics Aging* 9, no. 3 (2006): 190–194.

9. M. S. Garfinkel, H. R. Schumacher Jr., et al., "Evaluation of a yoga based regimen for treatment of osteoarthritis of the hands," *Journal of Rheumatology* 21, no. 12 (December 1994): 2341–2343. M. Garfinkel, "Yoga as a complementary therapy," *Geriatrics Aging* 9, no. 3 (2006): 190–194. S. L. Kolasinski, A. G. Tsai, et al., "Iyengar yoga for treating symptoms of osteoarthritis of the knees: A pilot study," *Journal of Alternative and Complementary Medicine* 11, no. 4 (August 2005): 689–693.

10. M. S. Garfinkel, H. R. Schumacher Jr., et al., "Evaluation of a yoga based regimen for treatment of osteoarthritis of the hands," *Journal of Rheumatology* 21, no. 12 (December 1994): 2341–2343. M. Garfinkel, "Yoga as a complementary therapy," *Geriatrics Aging* 9, no. 3 (2006): 190–194. S. L. Kolasinski, A. G. Tsai, et al., "Iyengar yoga for treating symptoms of osteoarthritis of the knees: A pilot study," *Journal of Alternative and Complementary Medicine* 11, no. 4 (August 2005): 689–693. M. Garfinkel and H. R. Schumacher Jr., "Yoga," *Rheumatic Diseases Clinics of North America* 26, no. 1 (February 2000): 125–132, x. M. S. Garfinkel, H. R. Schumacher Jr., et al., "Evaluation of a yoga based regimen for treatment of osteoarthritis of the hands," *Journal of Rheumatology* 21, no. 12 (December 1994): 2341. I. Haslock, R. Monro, et al., "Measuring the effects of yoga in rheumatoid arthritis," *British Journal of Rheumatology* 33, no. 8 (August 1994): 787–788.

11. S. Cooper, J. Oborne, et al., "Effect of two breathing exercises (Buteyko and pranayama) in asthma: A randomised controlled trial," *Thorax* 58, no. 8 (August 2003): 674–679. S. C. Jain, A. Uppal, et al., "A study of response pattern of non-insulin dependent diabetes to yoga therapy," *Diabetes Research and Clinical Practice* 19 (1993): 69–74.

12. S. Telles, B. H. Hanumanthaiah, et al., "Plasticity of motor control systems

demonstrated by yoga training," *Indian Journal of Physiological Pharmacology* 38, no. 2 (April 1994): 143–144.

13. S. W. Lazar, C. E. Kerr, et al., "Meditation experience is associated with increased cortical thickness," *Neuroreport* 16, no. 17 (November 2005): 1893–1897.

14. C. Peng, I. C. Henry, et al., "Heart rate dynamics during three forms of meditation," *International Journal of Cardiology* 95, no. 1 (May 2004): 19–27.

15. G. R. Deckro, K. M. Ballinger, et al., "The evaluation of a mind/body intervention to reduce psychological distress and perceived stress in college students," *Journal of American College Health* 50, no. 6 (May 2002): 281–287. R. P. Brown and P. L. Gerberg, "Sudarshan Kriya yogic breathing in the treatment of stress, anxiety, and depression: Part I—Neurophysiologic model," *Journal of Alternative and Complementary Medicine* 11, no. 1 (February 2005): 189–201. Erratum in: *Journal of Alternative and Complementary Medicine* 11, no. 2 (April 2005): 383–384.

16. M. DiBenedetto, K. E. Innes, et al., "Effect of a gentle Iyengar yoga program on gait in the elderly: An exploratory study," *Archives of Physical Medicine and Rehabilitation* 86 (September 2005): 1830–1837.

17. P. Raghuraj and S. Telles, "Effect of yoga-based and forced uninostril breathing on the autonomic nervous system," *Perceptual and Motor Skills* 96, no. 1 (February 2003): 79–80.

18. K. A. Williams, J. Petronis, et al., "Effect of Iyengar yoga therapy for chronic low back pain," *Pain* 115, nos. 1–2 (May 2005): 107–117. D. C. Cherkin, J. Erro, et al., "Comparing yoga, exercise, and a self-care book for chronic low back pain: A randomized trial," *Annals of Internal Medicine* 143 (2005): 849–856.

19. A. L. Williams, P. A. Selwyn, et al., "A randomized controlled trial of meditation and massage effects on quality of life in people with late-stage disease: A pilot study," *Journal of Palliative Medicine* 5 (October 2005): 939–952.

20. S. Cooper, J. Oborne, et al., "Effect of two breathing exercises (Buteyko and pranayama) in asthma: A randomised controlled trial," *Thorax* 58, no. 8 (August 2003): 674–679. G. R. Deckro, K. M. Ballinger, et al., "The evaluation of a mind/body intervention to reduce psychological distress and perceived stress in college students," *Journal of American College Health* 50, no. 6 (May 2002): 281–287.

21. L. Long, A. Huntley, and E. Ernst, "Which complementary and alternative therapies benefit which conditions? A survey of the opinions of 223 professional organizations," *Complementary Therapies in Medicine* 9, no. 3 (September 2001): 178–185.

22. *Hatha Yoga Pradipika*, chapter IV, verse 30, quoted in B. K. S. Iyengar, *Light on Yoga* (New York: Schocken Books, 1966), p. 45.

23. T. S. Elliot, *The Waste Land: A Norton Critical Edition*, edited by Michael North and Werner Sollors (New York: W. W. Norton, 2000).

24. Georg Feuerstein, *The Deeper Dimension of Yoga* (Boston: Shambala Publications, 2003), p. 349.

25. Ibid.

26. Sally Kempton, *The Heart of Meditation: Pathways to a Deeper Experience* (South Fallsburg, N.Y.: SYDA Foundation, 2002), p. 6.

27. Ibid., p. 20.

28. A. Cushman, "New Light on Yoga," *Yoga Journal* (July/August 1999): 44–49.

CHAPTER 3

1. J. P. Vedel and J. Mouillac-Baudevin, "Etude fonctionnelle du controle de l'activite des fibres fusimotrices dynamiques et statiques par les formations reticulees mesencephalique, pontique et bulbaire chez le chat," *Experimental Brain Research* 9 (1969): 325–345. R. Granit and B. Holmgren, "Two pathways from brain stem to gamma ventral horn cells," *Acta Physiologica Scandinavica* 35 (1955): 93–108. R. Granit, *Receptors and Sensory Perception* (New Haven: Yale University Press, 1955). P. H. Ellaway and J. R. Trott, "Autogenetic reflex action onto gamma motoneurons by stretch to triceps surae in the decerebrated cat," *Journal of Physiology* (*London*) 276 (1978): 49–66. V. S. Gurfinkel, M. I. Lipshits, et al., "The state of *stretch reflex* during quiet standing in man," *Progress in Brain Research* 44 (1976): 473–486. S. Gilman, J. S. Leiberman, and L. A. Marco, "Spinal mechanisms underlying the effects of unilateral ablation of areas 4 and 6 in monkeys," *Brain* 97 (1974): 49–64.

2. J. P. Vedel and J. Mouillac-Baudevin, "Etude fonctionnelle du controle de l'activite des fibres fusimotrices dynamiques et statiques par les formations reticulees mesencephalique, pontique et bulbaire chez le chat," *Experimental Brain Research* 9 (1969): 325–345. R. Granit and B. Holmgren, "Two pathways from brain stem to gamma ventral horn cells," *Acta Physiologica Scandinavica* 35 (1955): 93–108. P. H. Ellaway and J. R. Trott, "Autogenetic reflex action onto gamma motoneurons by stretch to triceps surae in the decerebrated cat," *Journal of Physiology* (*London*) 276 (1978): 49–66. V. S. Gurfinkel, M. I. Lipshits, et al., "The state of *stretch reflex* during quiet standing in man," *Progress in Brain Research* 44 (1976): 473–486.

3. J. P. Vedel and J. Mouillac-Baudevin, "Etude fonctionnelle du controle de l'activite des fibres fusimotrices dynamiques et statiques par les formations

reticulees mesencephalique, pontique et bulbaire chez le chat," *Experimental Brain Research* 9 (1969): 325–345.

4. J. P. Vedel and J. Mouillac-Baudevin, "Etude fonctionnelle du controle de l'activite des fibres fusimotrices dynamiques et statiques par les formations reticulees mesencephalique, pontique et bulbaire chez le chat," *Experimental Brain Research* 9 (1969): 325–345. P. H. Ellaway and J. R. Trott, "Autogenetic reflex action onto gamma motoneurons by stretch to triceps surae in the decerebrated cat," *Journal of Physiology* (*London*) 276 (1978): 49–66. V. S. Gurfinkel, M. I. Lipshits, et al., "The state of *stretch reflex* during quiet standing in man," *Progress in Brain Research* 44 (1976): 473–486.

5. J. P. Vedel and J. Mouillac-Baudevin, "Etude fonctionnelle du controle de l'activite des fibres fusimotrices dynamiques et statiques par les formations reticulees mesencephalique, pontique et bulbaire chez le chat," *Experimental Brain Research* 9 (1969): 325–345. R. Granit and B. Holmgren, "Two pathways from brain stem to gamma ventral horn cells," *Acta Physiologica Scandinavica* 35 (1955): 93–108. P. H. Ellaway and J. R. Trott, "Autogenetic reflex action onto gamma motoneurons by stretch to triceps surae in the decerebrated cat," *Journal of Physiology* (*London*) 276 (1978): 49–66. V. S. Gurfinkel, M. I. Lipshits, et al., "The state of *stretch reflex* during quiet standing in man," *Progress in Brain Research* 44 (1976): 473–486.

6. R. Granit, *Receptors and Sensory Perception* (New Haven: Yale University Press, 1955).

7. J. P. Vedel and J. Mouillac-Baudevin, "Etude fonctionnelle du controle de l'activite des fibres fusimotrices dynamiques et statiques par les formations reticulees mesencephalique, pontique et bulbaire chez le chat," *Experimental Brain Research* 9 (1969): 325–345. R. Granit and B. Holmgren, "Two pathways from brain stem to gamma ventral horn cells," *Acta Physiologica Scandinavica* 35 (1955): 93–108.

8. L. C. Junqueira and J. Carneiro, *Basic Histology*, 10th ed. (New York: McGraw-Hill, 2003), p. 136.

9. M. Garfinkel, H. R. Schumacher, et al., "Effect of joint motion on experimental calcium pyrophosphate dehydrated crystal induced arthritis," *Journal of Rheumatology* 17 (1990): 644–655. M. Garfinkel, "Yoga as a complementary therapy," *Geriatrics Aging* 9, no. 3 (2006): 190–194. M. Garfinkel and H. R. Schumacher, "Yoga," *Rheumatic Diseases Clinics of North America* 26, no. 1 (February 2000): 125–132, x.

10. L. C. Junqueira and J. Carneiro, *Basic Histology*, 10th ed. (New York: McGraw-Hill, 2003), p. 136.

11. G. W. Thorn, R. D. Adams, et al., *Harrison's Principles of Internal Medicine*, 8th ed. (New York: McGraw-Hill, 1977), p. 2071.

12. G. W. Thorn, R. D. Adams, et al., *Harrison's Principles of Internal Medicine*, 8th ed. (New York: McGraw-Hill, 1977), p. 2071. G. Tardif, J. P. Pelletier, et al., "Differential regulation of the bone morphogenic protein antagonist chordin in human normal and osteoarthritic chondrocytes," *Annals of the Rheumatic Diseases* 65, no. 2 (February 2006): 261–264. M. Renoux, P. Hilliquin, et al., "Cellular activation products in osteoarthritis synovial fluid," *International Journal of Clinical Pharmacology Research* 15, no. 4 (1995): 135–138. K. Masuko-Hongo, T. Sato, and K. Nishioka, "Chemokines differentially induce matrix metalloproteinase-3 and prostaglandin E2 in human articular chondrocytes," *Clinical and Experimental Rheumatology* 23, no. 1 (January–February 2005): 57–61. J. A. Hannafin, E. A. Attia, et al., "Effect of cyclic strain and plating matrix on cell proliferation and integrin expression by ligament fibroblasts," *Journal of Orthopaedic Research* 24, no. 2 (February 2006): 149–158.

13. G. Tardif, J. P. Pelletier, et al., "Differential regulation of the bone morphogenic protein antagonist chordin in human normal and osteoarthritic chondrocytes," *Annals of the Rheumatic Diseases* 65, no. 2 (February 2006): 261–264. M. Renoux, P. Hilliquin, et al., "Cellular activation products in osteoarthritis synovial fluid," *International Journal of Clinical Pharmacology Research* 15, no. 4 (1995): 135–138. K. Masuko-Hongo, T. Sato, and K. Nishioka, "Chemokines differentially induce matrix metalloproteinase-3 and prostaglandin E2 in human articular chondrocytes," *Clinical and Experimental Rheumatology* 23, no. 1 (January–February 2005): 57–61.

14. C. J. Wolff and M. W. Salter, "Neuronal plasticity: Increasing the gain in pain," *Science* 288 (2000): 1765–1768.

15. H. Ollar and P. Cesaro, "Pharmacology of neuropathic pain," *Clinical Neuropharmacology* 18 (1995): 391–404.

16. These studies are particularly relevant to yoga therapy:
    S. Gilman, J. S. Leiberman, and L. A. Marco, "Spinal mechanisms underlying the effects of unilateral ablation of areas 4 and 6 in monkeys," *Brain* 97 (1974): 49–64.
    M. Garfinkel, H. R. Schumacher, et al., "Effect of joint motion on experimental calcium pyrophosphate dehydrated crystal induced arthritis," *Journal of Rheumatology* 17 (1990): 644–655.
    M. Garfinkel, "Yoga as a complementary therapy," *Geriatrics Aging* 9, no. 3 (2006): 190–194.
    M. Garfinkel and H. R. Schumacher, "Yoga," *Rheumatic Diseases Clinics of North America* 26, no. 1 (February 2000): 125–132, x.
    R. P. Brown and P. L. Gerbarg, "Sudarshan Kriya yogic breathing in the treatment of stress, anxiety, and depression: Part I—Neurophysiologic model," *Journal of Alternative and Complementary Medicine* 11, no. 1 (February 2005): 189–201.

Erratum in: *Journal of Alternative and Complementary Medicine* 11, no. 2 (April 2005): 383–384.

D. C. Cherkin, J. Erro, et al., "Comparing yoga, exercise, and a self-care book for chronic low back pain: A randomized trial," *Annals of Internal Medicine* 143 (2005): 849–856.

S. Cooper, J. Oborne, et al., "Effect of two breathing exercises (Buteyko and pranayama) in asthma: A randomised controlled trial," *Thorax* 58, no. 8 (August 2003): 674–679.

G. R. Deckro, K. M. Ballinger, et al., "The evaluation of a mind/body intervention to reduce psychological distress and perceived stress in college students," *Journal of American College Health* 50, no. 6 (May 2002): 281–287.

M. DiBenedetto, K. E. Innes, et al., "Effect of a gentle Iyengar yoga program on gait in the elderly: An exploratory study," *Archives of Physical Medicine and Rehabilitation* 86 (September 2005): 1830–1837.

L. M. Fishman and C. A. Ardman, *Relief Is in the Stretch: End Back Pain through Yoga* (New York: W. W. Norton, 2005).

L. Fishman, C. Konnot, and A. Polesin. "Headstand for rotator cuff: *sirsasana* or surgery," *Journal of the International Association of Yoga Therapists* 16 (October 2006).

L. M. Fishman and C. Konnoth, "Role of headstand in the management of rotator cuff syndrome," *American Journal of Physical Medicine and Rehabilitation* 83, no. 3 (March 2004): 8, Abstract.

M. S. Garfinkel, H. R. Schumacher Jr., et al., "Evaluation of a yoga based regimen for treatment of osteoarthritis of the hands," *Journal of Rheumatology* 21, no. 12 (December 1994): 2341–2343.

I. Haslock, R. Monro, et al., "Measuring the effects of yoga in rheumatoid arthritis," *British Journal of Rheumatology* 33, no. 8 (August 1994): 787–788.

S. C. Jain, A. Uppal, et al., "A study of response pattern of non-insulin dependent diabetes to yoga therapy," *Diabetes Research and Clinical Practice* 19 (1993): 69–74.

S. L. Kolasinski, A. G. Tsai, et al., "Iyengar yoga for treating symptoms of osteoarthritis of the knees: A pilot study," *Journal of Alternative and Complementary Medicine* 11, no. 4 (August 2005): 689–693.

S. W. Lazar, C. E. Kerr, et al., "Meditation experience is associated with increased cortical thickness," *Neuroreport* 16, no. 17 (November 2005): 1893–1897.

B. S. Oken, S. Kishiyama, et al., "Randomized controlled trial of yoga and exercise in multiple sclerosis," *Neurology* 62, no. 11 (June 8, 2004): 2058–2064.

C. Peng, I. C. Henry, et al., "Heart rate dynamics during three forms of meditation," *International Journal of Cardiology* 95, no. 1 (May 2004): 19–27.

P. Raghuraj and S. Telles, "Effect of yoga-based and forced uninostril breathing on the autonomic nervous system," *Perceptual and Motor Skills* 96, no. 1 (February 2003): 79–80.

S. Telles, B. H. Hanumanthaiah, et al., "Plasticity of motor control systems demonstrated by yoga training," *Indian Journal of Physiological Pharmacology* 38, no. 2 (April 1994): 143–144.

J. Wolff, *The Law of Bone Remodeling* (Berlin: Springer, 1986) (translation of the German 1892 edition).

K. A. Williams, J. Petronis, et al., "Effect of Iyengar yoga therapy for chronic low back pain," *Pain* 115, nos. 1–2 (May 2005): 107–117.

CHAPTER 7

1. *Medical Care* 41, no. 12 (2003): 1367–1375. [Data Source: 1997 National Hospital Discharge Survey (NHDS)]

CHAPTER 13

1. Renee Cailliet, *The Feet and Ankles* (Philadelphia: W. B. Saunders, 1986).

2. Ibid.

RESOURCES

Yoga Teachers and Therapists

Listings of Anusara-trained teachers   *www.anusara.com*
Listings of Iyengar-trained teachers   *www.iynaus.org*
Integral Yoga Teachers Association   *www.iyta.org*

International Association of Yoga Therapists
115 S. McCormick Street
Suite 3
Prescott, AZ 86303
Phone: 928–541–0004
Fax: 928–541–0182
Email: *mail@iayt.org*
Web site: *www.iayt.org*

Yoga Alliance
7801 Old Branch Avenue
Suite 400
Clinton, MD 20735
Phone: 877–964–2255
Fax: 301–868–7909
Web site: *www.yogaalliance.org*

Yoga Information Web Sites

Yoga Research and Education Foundation   *www.yref.org*
Yoga Journal   *www.yogajournal.com*
Yoga + Joyful Living magazine   *www.himalayaninstitute.org/yogaplus*
Yoga for osteoporosis   *www.sciatica.org*
Yoga props   *www.huggermugger.com*
    www.toolsforyoga.com

Books

HATHA YOGA THERAPY

Fishman, Loren, and Carol Ardman. *Cure Back Pain with Yoga*. New York: W. W. Norton, 2005. Yoga for back pain by diagnosis.

Fishman, Loren, and Eric Small. *Yoga for Multiple Sclerosis*. New York: Demos Medical Publishing, 2007. Restorative and problem-directed sections applicable to several neurological diseases.

Iyengar, B. K. S. *Light on Yoga*. New York: Schocken Books, many editions. The classic modern text with over six hundred pictures.

Lasater, Judith. *Relax and Renew: Restful Yoga for Stressful Times*. Berkeley, Calif.: Rodmell Press, 1995. The authoritative book on restorative yoga.

McCall, Timothy. *Yoga as Medicine*. San Francisco: The Yoga Journal, 2007. Excellent all-round summary of yoga therapy from leading experts, including Dr. McCall.

Schatz, Mary Pullig. *Back Care Basics: A Doctor's Gentle Yoga Program for Back and Neck Pain Relief*. Berkeley, Calif.: Rodmell Press, 1995. A beneficial program.

Sparrowe, Linda, and Patricia Walden. *The Woman's Book of Yoga and Health: A Lifelong Guide to Wellness*. Boston: Shambhala, 2002. Compendious and safe.

PHILOSOPHY AND MEDITATION

Feuerstein, Georg. *The Deeper Dimension of Yoga: Theory and Practice*. Boston: Shambhala, 2003. A book of short essays on many topics central to yoga.

Iyengar, B. K. S. *Light on the Yoga Sutras of Patanjali*. London: Thorsons, 1996.

Kempton, Sally. *The Heart of Meditation: Pathways to a Deeper Experience*. South Fallsburg, N.Y.: SYDA Foundation, 2002. Excellent introduction to meditation that goes quite deep.

Mascaró, Juan (trans.). *The Bhagavad Gita*. Baltimore: Penguin Books, 1962.

Shearer, Alistair (trans.). *The Yoga Sutras of Patanjali*. New York: Bell Tower, 1982.

Taimni, I. K. *The Science of Yoga*. Wheaton, Ill.: Quest Books, Theosophical Publishing House, 1972. The Yoga sutra in Sanskrit with transliteration, translation, and commentary.

Northport-East Northport Public Library

MAY 2008

To view your patron record from a computer, click on
the Library's homepage: **www.nenpl.org**

You may:

- request an item be placed on hold
- renew an item that is overdue
- view titles and due dates checked out on your card
- view your own outstanding fines

151 Laurel Avenue
Northport, NY 11768
631-261-6930